ON BECOMING A HEALER

On Becoming a Healer

The Journey from Patient Care to Caring about Your Patients

SAUL J. WEINER, MD

JOHNS HOPKINS UNIVERSITY PRESS | *Baltimore*

© 2020 Johns Hopkins University Press
All rights reserved. Published 2020
Printed in the United States of America on acid-free paper
9 8 7 6 5 4 3 2 1

Johns Hopkins University Press
2715 North Charles Street
Baltimore, Maryland 21218-4363
www.press.jhu.edu

Library of Congress Cataloging-in-Publication Data

Names: Weiner, Saul J., author.
Title: On becoming a healer : the journey from patient care to caring about your
    patients / Saul J. Weiner, MD.
Description: Baltimore : Johns Hopkins University Press, 2020. | Includes
    bibliographical references and index.
Identifiers: LCCN 2019031190 | ISBN 9781421437811 (paperback ; alk. paper) |
    ISBN 9781421437828 (ebook)
Subjects: MESH: Physician-Patient Relations | Education, Medical
Classification: LCC R727.3 | NLM W 62 | DDC 610.69/6—dc23
LC record available at https://lccn.loc.gov/2019031190

A catalog record for this book is available from the British Library.

*Special discounts are available for bulk purchases of this book. For
more information, please contact Special Sales at specialsales@press.jhu.edu.*

Johns Hopkins University Press uses environmentally friendly book materials,
including recycled text paper that is composed of at least 30 percent post-consumer
waste, whenever possible.

For Simon

CONTENTS

This book would not have been conceivable without the inspiration and profound influence of Dr. Simon Auster, a retired family medicine physician, psychiatrist, and educator, to whom it is dedicated. During our many years of conversation, I took copious notes, which have been an invaluable resource. Having suffered a stroke, he is no longer able to read on his own. However, throughout the writing process I often read to him sections of chapters when I needed help. Most important, like many others touched by him, through our relationship I have learned what it is to be healed.

On Becoming a Healer also builds on *Listening for What Matters,* coauthored with my distinguished colleague and close friend Alan Schwartz, PhD. That empirical work describes more than a decade of research based on thousands of audio recordings of medical encounters, with a focus on the physician's attention (or lack thereof) to the life challenges of their patients when planning their care. Alan, along with a small cadre of research assistants—Naomi Ashley, Amy Binns-Calvey, Benjamin Kass, Brendan Kelly, and Gunjan Sharma—enabled that body of work to come to fruition. *On Becoming a Healer* stands on these two pillars: the wisdom of Simon and the collective insight and commitment of our team.

In addition, I am grateful to premedical students, medical students, residents, and attending physicians who volunteered to provide feedback on individual chapters, including Ahmeed Aleem, Jillian Caldwell, Camila Castellanos, Pyone David, Benjamin Goldenberg, Anna Gramelspacher, Jacob Grand, Mary Hardin, Augustin Joseph, David Kasjanski, Wasan Kumar, Jessica Lee, Kevin Lee, Caitlin Lopes, Maggie Mass, Wenyu Pan, Agata Parfieniuk, Raj Patel, Jorge Ramallo,

Hilary Renaldy, Steven Rothschild, Michelle Sheena, Chris Viamontes, Maya Viner, Jennifer Vu, and Chase Westra. Their helpful feedback from a reader's perspective guided my final revisions.

I also acknowledge the US Department of Veterans Affairs—particularly the Center of Innovation for Complex Chronic Healthcare, directed by Frances Weaver these past ten years, and based at Hines VA Hospital and Jesse Brown VA Medical Centers—and the University of Illinois at Chicago, the two organizations where I've concurrently spent my professional career. The former has funded much of the research described, and together they have provided the setting for many of the anecdotes I relate, along with those from my medical school and residency training days. Finally, I'd like to acknowledge the Institute for Practice and Provider Performance Improvement (I3PI) and its supporters, particularly the Robert Wood Johnson Foundation, for enabling Alan, me, and our team to utilize unannounced standardized patients, or "secret shoppers," to observe health care delivery in the private sector, leading to many of the observations in this book. I would like to emphasize that both the good and the bad incidents were selected to illustrate underlying themes that are broadly generalizable, not because I think they reflect particular characteristics of the institutions and settings where I've happened to train, practice, and teach medicine or conduct research.

A work as personal and life-spanning as this one draws on too many conversations, friendships, and shared experiences to acknowledge all who contributed by challenging me, sharing an idea, or simply showing the way by example. Special thanks, however, to my wife, Suzanne Griffel, for her meticulous editing of the manuscript, which went far beyond grammar and spelling checks to spotting inconsistencies, lapses in logic, and so forth. In addition, she and my daughter, Karen, lovingly put up with me when I was at less than my best—particularly when trying to meet deadlines—for which I am especially grateful.

ON BECOMING A HEALER

Introduction

L IKE MANY aspiring physicians, I felt called to a career in medicine yet knew little about what I was getting into. My first medical school interview was with an amiable rheumatologist in a charmless office at a large, run-down, urban hospital, on a corridor tucked behind an industrial-sized kitchen. As I came in the main entrance, wearing a new suit, I noticed the peculiar corrosive smell of hospital disinfectant, saw elderly patients on gurneys, and felt sad and confused inside. At the time, I couldn't articulate why. The interview was relaxed, friendly, and seemed to go well, which put me in a better mood. Getting to this point had been a long and difficult road for me, so I had every reason to be excited. As I headed home, I was able to push out of my consciousness the unease—bordering on dread—that I'd experienced before the interview. But I sensed it would return.

I'd actually had more experience with health care delivery than many aspiring physicians. In high school, I trained and worked as an emergency medical technician on a rural volunteer ambulance squad. I once performed CPR on a farmer who had aspirated chewing tobacco, pushing hard on his chest while trying to keep my balance in the back of the van as the driver, with sirens blaring, whisked us to the emergency department. Shortly after we got there, the man was pronounced dead. I wondered if maybe I could have saved him if I had known more. In college I observed and studied health care in the developing world, spending the summer after my junior year shadowing physicians at clinics and hospitals in Nepal. Throughout, I strategized about what I needed to do to become a doctor. Getting into medical school became an obsession.

Yet, once on the threshold of entering the profession, I wondered silently if I was making a mistake. What hung over me was the feeling that I didn't know if I would be happy with my chosen vocation. I recalled going to see my pediatrician in high school, in a nice office where he saw kid after kid coming in with colds and for school physicals, and feeling a disconnect between what I imagined his job was like and the excitement of being a doctor. His demeanor, which seemed fatherly but distant, may have contributed to my misgivings. It was a trepidation that felt shameful to articulate, as I had already embraced the identity. After all, being a physician is supposed to be a "privilege," as one acquires the knowledge and skills to cure disease and alleviate suffering and becomes privy to the intimate lives of patients. While I could exude confidence and enthusiasm about where I was headed, inside I felt like someone who sensed they might be marrying the wrong person.

It's taken me years to understand the source of the ambivalence I felt at the time. Joy in medicine requires more than idealistic aspirations; it requires a capacity to see past the "otherness" that separates the well from the sick, the old from the young, the professional in a white coat from the disheveled patient in a hospital gown, and fully embrace their shared humanity. And at that stage in my career, I didn't have that capacity.

When one is unable to bridge the divide between doctor and patient, medicine becomes a career rather than a calling. Medicine as a career is about advancement, status, fitting in, making money, finding job security, and working reasonable hours. For some it's also about the intellectual rewards of learning new procedures, guidelines, and research related to patient care. In addition, most physicians enjoy the human interaction with patients and consider it a central part of their professional identity. But how many are capable of relationships that are mutually nourishing?

Few are, it seems. The irony that premeds are often the last people you'd want to turn to in a time of need became evident to me in college when I first learned about the selection process for a peer-to-peer support program. The campus counseling center ran an off-hours service where students could meet with other students to talk about loneliness, depression, relationship problems, or anything else on their minds. At the orientation meeting, premeds were cautioned against applying for the purpose of buttressing their résumés. Such careerism was widely recognized. The prospect of would-be physicians serving as peer counselors was something people joked about. Premeds were satirized as the students who would break your pencil during a chemistry exam if given the chance.

What are the ideal characteristics of someone with whom to share personal matters? The peer counseling program looked for certain qualities. First is unselfconsciously giving others one's undivided attention, without predisposition to making assumptions, and without pretension that one is somehow superior. In the screening interviews, the program's leaders sought students who were comfortable acknowledging and talking about their own problems. A mentor, Simon Auster, who came to play a central role in my development as a physician, described those behaviors, collectively, as "a capacity to openly and fully engage." One could say they were looking for people who are "real."

The second characteristic is that they have interpersonal boundary clarity, meaning they can distinguish what's them from what's the other person. When you talk with someone about your problems, you want to know that they are not confusing their needs and wants with yours. Parents often frustrate their young adult children, for instance, when they regard them as extensions of themselves, coloring the advice they give. A young woman trying to make it as a writer is not going to get good counsel from a father who is dismissive and tells her she should go to law school, as he envisions her taking over his practice. A patient considering whether to stop chemotherapy near the end of life is not going to get good counsel from a physician who believes that—as one of my research oncology professors put it—"everyone should die on a protocol." Whose interests are these individuals representing? Without respecting—or even recognizing—interpersonal boundaries, they disregard others' values and preferences when they differ from their own.

Engagement and boundary clarity are the yin and yang of every healing interaction. If one is missing, the other may do more harm than good. To engage without boundary clarity is intrusive. When an angry couple lose their tempers and yell at one another, they are most definitely engaging, but without respect for boundaries, the interaction is more likely to wound than heal. Conversely, maintaining boundaries without engagement fosters alienation. Acting friendly while not really being interested is a prevalent aspect of American culture that does little to alleviate loneliness. At the supermarket checkout counter, when the cashier asks, "How are you today?" and you respond without thinking, "Fine, thank you," no boundaries are crossed, but neither is there a meaningful connection. In the doctor's office, the vulnerable patient seeking human connection may attempt to engage, but all too often the physician is on autopilot, focused on writing their notes, as in: "So sorry to hear about your loss. . . . Any bowel or bladder problems?" There is a sad pattern here: In our personal lives we are prone to engage without respecting boundaries, and in our professional lives it's the other way around—that is, we maintain boundaries but often fail to engage. Neither is healing.

Unfortunately, those entering medicine often have trouble with both. Many come from family and educational environments where boundaries are crossed. They have experienced hurt and humiliation, which makes them habitually guarded. In non-intimate relationships they learn to skillfully keep a distance: in lieu of engagement, they acquire a professional persona that is unassailable but somewhat heartless and insincere. While primarily self-protective, it is also secondarily protective of their patients. If you are not clear about boundaries, it is probably better not to engage, as you may unwittingly say things that are hurtful. Pleasantries and small talk are preferable to disrespectful interaction.

Joy in medicine, however, does require open and full engagement with a wide range of individuals, often from very different backgrounds and life experiences. When I walked into that hospital for my first medical school interview, I had not yet learned how to engage in the professional sphere. When I gazed at an elderly, ill woman in a wheelchair, it never occurred to me that she and I were on the same journey called life, except that she was further along. When I saw a homeless man, I didn't appreciate that this was a person who had mastered a whole set of survival skills that I knew nothing about. Seeing patients as "other," I held them at arm's length. This generated cognitive dissonance: in theory I valued connecting with patients and saw it as an attraction to medicine, but in reality I didn't know how.

Medical training makes it difficult to confront the emotional issues that often surface in young adulthood. College is over, yet school is harder and more regimented than ever. Persevering requires single-minded focus. Inner pain is suppressed and self-awareness underdeveloped. Like many, I came to medicine with both strengths and challenges. I had wanted to be a doctor for years but struggled with a learning disability that made science courses particularly onerous. I took chemistry during the summer before college prior to matriculating. Working nearly every waking hour, seeking out the teaching assistant daily for tutoring, I earned a C. Then I took it again, this time freshman year when it went on my transcript, and managed to get a B. I got okay grades in the rest of my premedical courses by working really hard to digest just enough knowledge to make it through most of my exams.

During my first year of medical school, I felt especially alone. Whatever strengths I had were not the ones valued by the institution. After a few months I figured out how to play the game—at least well enough to pass exams. It involved memorizing the professors' handouts even if I didn't understand what I was memorizing, reading concise outline-style review books, and then taking lots of old practice tests. This required skipping lectures, which I couldn't follow anyway, to free up the time. While an effective survival strategy, it was also demoralizing, as I did not feel anything approaching a sense of competency, let alone mastery. It felt more like fakery. It occurred to me that some others were probably in a similar boat, but it also seemed as if quite a few people were getting along just fine.

I began to think that the particular qualities that characterize a good physician may not be the same as those required of a first- or second-year medical school student, but that was not much comfort at the time. Struggling through courses had a corrosive effect on my self-esteem. Looking for relief, I became preoccupied with a young woman with whom I had shared an on-and-off relationship starting in undergraduate school. I felt that if she wanted to be my girlfriend, that validated my worth. At the same time, I recognized that we were not compatible or, at least, that our dynamic was not good for me. During the brief period when the relationship was back on, I felt euphoric, and when it was off, I attributed all of my misery to that loss. One evening I found myself pacing the narrow hallway on the first floor of my townhouse, sobbing so loudly that the neighbors called and asked me to come over. They were a couple in their fifties. He could be brusque, as I had learned early on: the first day I moved in, I dragged a washer-dryer I had purchased across our shared lawn, flattening the grass, and he came out and yelled at me. But we had since started to get along, after some friendlier chance interactions. I've not forgotten their act of kindness—summoning me to join them for drinks and a card game, no questions asked—at a time when I really needed it.

When a Caring Mentor Reaches Out

It was at this low point that someone uniquely capable of helping me stepped in. My parents had designated Simon Auster as my godfather shortly after my birth. We were already close before I entered medical school, but only as close as I was capable of being at the time, owing— as I came to appreciate years later—to a limited capacity to trust. Simon, who was trained as both a family medicine physician and a psychiatrist, said to me on one of our occasional weekend phone calls, "You know, Saul, I think it might be helpful if you and I started to talk regularly." I accepted the invitation and entered what would be a combination of therapy and mentoring that would last decades. We've spoken nearly every Saturday for thirty years.

Simon encouraged my desire to form personal connections with patients and families at a fundamentally human level rather than to adopt the persona of a physician—in other words, he promoted engagement.

He also helped me set appropriate boundaries, such that my unscripted self was therapeutic rather than unfocused or self-indulgent in patient encounters. This sort of emotional support and guidance enabled a trajectory that was likely quite different from that of most of my colleagues.

Most are taught what is often referred to as "good bedside manner." Instead of learning to keep it personal, medical students acquire a set of scripted behaviors, that is, "manners." I remember in my second year of medical school conducting a practice medical interview while my peers watched and a physician faculty member observed and took notes. I lost points for forgetting to sit at eye level with the patient and reach out sympathetically to touch her on the arm when I was supposed to. The problem was that I was too absorbed in the conversation to remember these "rapport building tactics." I was able to articulate my frustration to Simon during one of our Saturday morning calls when I said, "Bedside manner seems to be a set of rules for people who don't know how to care."

Another example of the socialization process is from my pediatric clerkship, a year later. I was assigned to a team caring for a fourteen-year-old girl with lupus, who I'll call Lorrie. An array of specialists visited Lorrie daily, arriving at her bedside at different times and not communicating much with each other. This was a source of frustration for her parents. I recall meeting with them several times in a small, private room where they poured out anxieties and concerns about her care. I was able to schedule a meeting of all the doctors to arrive at a plan. While I formed a connection with her parents, I don't recall spending much time with Lorrie. Her friends came and went as she endured kidney biopsies, dialysis, and episodes of internal bleeding. At that stage in my life I was more comfortable relating to adults than to an adolescent girl.

At the end of the rotation I received an evaluation from the director of the pediatrics clerkship in which she expressed concern about my relationship with Lorrie's family. Her evaluation was based on feedback she got from the residents I worked with every day. She wrote that my level of "overinvolvement was likely, if it continued, to lead to burnout." She also raised concerns that I was overstepping my bounds as a medical student, acting as if I were the senior doctor in my interactions with the parents. For me, however, my role in Lorrie's care had sustained me. It was hard and sad at times, but I felt useful and connected. Also, rather than supplanting a more senior doctor, I felt I was filling a void. No one else was coordinating Lorrie's care. Nevertheless, the feedback I got felt humiliating and left me with doubts. I wondered if I had been some sort of an imposter who took advantage of Lorrie's parents' vulnerabilities to feed some inner need for validation. That was the message I was getting. Talking with Simon provided a critical counterpoint. He challenged me to reach inside and answer for myself whether I thought my behaviors were appropriate or not, so that I could become my own compass. Over time that led to greater self-trust.

Some months later I heard that Lorrie had died. I don't recall reaching out to the parents or sending a note of condolence. I hope I did, but it wouldn't have been something we were taught to do. On the contrary, when you left a month "on service," you moved on. Decades later, as the father of a grown child, I feel anger at the disconnect between medical school teachers' fretting about a student's "overinvolvement" and the heartbreaking struggle of a family to keep their daughter alive, desperately dependent on an emotionally distant health care team.

Without someone to talk with about what I was going through during those years, I might have stopped engaging with patients. I might have become more like the residents who were uncomfortable with their "overly involved" medical student. Such a state of mind stunts personal growth, as the self retreats into a shell. Safely encased, the emerging physician adopts an assured manner of handling any situation, whether it be an angry parent or a struggling patient. But what they are doing is just that—"handling"—rather than engaging with another person who may be frightened or suffering, in need of real human connection. I recall my awe as a student of a particularly confident senior resident who effortlessly put out any fire. When called to the bedside of a disruptive patient on the psychiatry ward, he slipped in an IV, infused Haldol, and returned the patient to a state of medicated calm. When I related the encounter to Simon, he wondered out loud what we might have learned if we'd asked the patient what he was upset about instead. That got me thinking: is it okay to stick a needle in someone just because you are a doctor and you think you know what is best?

Questioning What You See

Over the years, it became increasingly apparent to me that physicians are remarkably incurious about the life circumstances and behaviors of their patients. When they don't take their medications correctly, we lecture them about how they have to do a better job rather that asking them what happened. When they get angry or anxious, doctors often get defensive or try to calm them down rather than first asking questions to better understand where their patient is coming from. To what extent does this lack of interest affect care?

I decided to explore that question after a particularly memorable patient encounter when I was a junior attending physician. Ms. Dawson (not her real name) showed up in the presurgery assessment clinic that I was staffing with a couple of residents whom I supervised. After seeing her first, one of them explained to me that Ms. Dawson was scheduled for bariatric surgery to treat her obesity. The resident presented the patient's medical history and test results, concluding that everything was in order for her to proceed to the operating room. As we headed into the exam room together, the resident offhandedly mentioned that "Ms. Dawson's looking forward to having the surgery so that she can better care of her son"—sharing the comment, it seemed, as further evidence that surgery was the right way to go. Before entering I asked, "What's wrong with him?" The resident shrugged and said, "I don't know," with a look that seemed to convey impatience. Perhaps she wondered why the son's health care problems mattered. After all, he wasn't our patient.

I could appreciate where she was coming from because I recalled that when I was in her shoes, I just couldn't seem to please my attendings by knowing enough. However prepared I was on hospital rounds in the mornings, they'd ask me for some obscure factoid about the patient to which I didn't have a response other than "I don't know." The blank stare I'd get left me feeling like I'd let them down. At the same time, I'd wonder why the information was relevant. I didn't ask, and they didn't tell me. I thought it might just be a game of one-upmanship.

When I asked Ms. Dawson about her son, I learned that he was a young man in his early twenties in the advanced stages of muscular dystrophy, with muscle atrophy and contractures. She was his sole caretaker, lifting him each time he needed to be transferred to his bath, bed, or a chair. She also parented a younger daughter and lived with an alcoholic husband. If she went ahead with the surgery, she wouldn't be able to do any heavy lifting for several weeks. While she'd considered how losing weight would ease caring for her son, she hadn't thought about the long recovery. Because she'd previously had her gallbladder out and had scar tissue in her abdomen, her surgery would require a large incision. This meant that if she lifted her son during the first month after the operation, she risked opening the surgical wound. Once all this came out in our discussion, Ms. Dawson canceled the procedure. She concluded it wasn't at all what she wanted or could tolerate at the time.

After seeing the consequences of disinterest in patients' life situations, I started to work with a research colleague named Alan Schwartz, who is a cognitive psychologist interested in how physicians make medical decisions. This was a time when studies were exposing high rates of medical error. A national report showed that between 50,000 and 100,000 people die in the United States each year because physicians prescribe the wrong drug or the wrong dose of the right drug, operate on the wrong limb, overlook necessary steps to prevent drug-resistant infections, and so forth. Each of these errors was given a name, such as "medication error," "diagnostic error," or "treatment error." I decided to call errors that occur because the physician doesn't know something critical about the patient's life situation "contextual errors." Sending Ms. Dawson to the operating room would have been a contextual error. And it could have had serious consequences. Out of an overriding need to care for her son, she might have had a major setback in wound healing if she'd lifted him before she was medically ready.

Alan and I have been studying contextual errors for over a decade.

Ascertaining whether a doctor is overlooking critical information about patients' life situations that is relevant to their care requires listening in on the visit. We've adopted two strategies: training actors to show up in doctors' offices with a concealed audio recorder while portraying patients who drop clues that they are facing a life challenge, and inviting real patients to record their visits. We then listen for whether the physician notices the clues, asks about them, and addresses contextual factors where feasible when planning care. Participating physicians have agreed not to know when they are interacting with a fake or real patient who is collecting data. Our book *Listening for What Matters: Avoiding Contextual Errors in Health Care* describes this work and what we learned.

What does contextualizing care have to do with engagement? I think it's fair to say that a physician who is missing clues that a patient is struggling with a life challenge that affects their care is probably not engaged in the interaction. To assess physician attention, we instructed one actor to sigh and say, "Boy it's been tough since I've lost my job" during dozens of visits portraying a patient whose asthma flared up when they could no longer afford an expensive brand-name medication. The actor was told not to reveal their financial problems unless asked. All too often distracted physicians would nod and respond to the comment, absentmindedly, with something like, "Sorry to hear that. . . . Do you have any allergies?" while they typed and looked at a screen. The minority of physicians who were giving the patient their full attention would ask, "How has it been tough?" and typically follow with, "Are you having trouble affording your medications?" When physicians were distracted, they tended to order more medications that the patient couldn't afford, as well as additional pointless tests and referrals. When they were engaged, they simply switched the patient to a less costly generic.

Remarkably, we discovered that contextualizing care doesn't lengthen the visit. The time spent learning about patients' life challenges was offset by time saved on the back end of the visit, by skipping unhelpful discussions regarding additional testing and medications that weren't warranted. These findings should be reassuring to physicians who worry that if they start delving into life issues as they pertain to care planning, it will take too long and they'll keep other patients waiting.

Doing research on physician-patient interaction has further inspired me to write this book, not only because we learned that contextualizing care need not be time-consuming but because it has measurable value: attention to the context of patients' lives favorably affects health care outcomes. We saw repeatedly, for instance, that patients who had diabetes were more likely to get control of their blood sugars if their physicians identified and worked with them to address underlying impediments to medication adherence than if these were overlooked. Discovering that these more substantive discussions don't even take longer was "icing on the cake," as it debunked the argument that physicians don't have time to form therapeutic human connections.

Physician, Heal Thyself

Why are doctors disengaged? One reason I hear is that they feel that asking personal questions is like "opening Pandora's box" and that they'll never get out of the exam room. As noted, research indicates that is not the case. Another possibility is that they don't have a lot of patience for human nature. I've seen how patients are subtly blamed for their problems with phrases like "she is noncompliant" or "he is drug seeking," when they are just being, well, human! Sadly, it seems that it is in those situations where patients are struggling the most that physicians are most inclined to keep them at bay. The dynamic isn't good for either party. Patients are left unsatisfied, and physicians become cynical and susceptible to burnout.

Medical students tend to adopt the same attitudes about patients and patient care. While I had someone to guide me during my medical education, few physicians-in-training are so fortunate. Without help finding their way, they are socialized to the norms of the profession, modeling their behavior on what they observe. I was fortunate to have someone challenge me to follow a different course. With Simon's unsentimental grounding, I came to see that doctors hide behind their white coats while patients want to connect with a real person who cares about them.

With Simon's mentorship I also learned that good doctors are comfortable not having all the answers, because they know the visit is not about them. They appreciate that if they take advantage of the opportunity to form human connections with their patients, those connections, combined with their expert knowledge of the health care system and what it can and cannot offer, will nearly always bring value to the patient. This perspective has guided me to engage with patients as who I am rather than to adopt a script, confident that doing so is best for both them and me. Admittedly, I don't think I could have acquired this self-trust on my own. It took coaching from someone who didn't hesitate to challenge me—and it took quite some time before I was fully receptive to being challenged. First I had to learn to trust Simon, and then, from there, I was gradually able to learn to trust myself.

While this book cannot substitute for one-on-one mentoring, it systematically lays out a number of ideas and concepts that took me years to appreciate. I've added questions at the end of each chapter to foster reflection and discussion. *On Becoming a Healer* speaks to those with an open heart who have not yet found a way to harness such a powerful resource in the service of healing.

Lessons for Living

Another reason I decided to write this book is that the lessons I learned from Simon have helped me outside of the medical setting as well. A former student of Simon's, who later became his physician, put it succinctly: "You practice medicine the way you live your life."

If this book has a single message, it's that you can't be remote and controlling with one set of people and a kind and thoughtful healer with others. Engaging with boundary clarity is a way of being in relation to other people that is intrinsically grounded in an appreciation of how we all share a common human experience, with vulnerabilities and interdependencies. No one escapes misfortune, illness, and death.

Nearly all rely on others for stability, security, and well-being. Living with this appreciation as a guide to action isn't just for professional healers. The most effective and contented managers, leaders, parents, teachers, and citizens are healers.

The impact of this book will depend largely on my gaining your trust that there is nothing exaggerated or romanticized here. That way, hopefully, if certain arguments don't initially make sense to you, you will give them serious reflection nonetheless. I do not sugarcoat aspects of my job that I find tedious and unrewarding. In the settings in which I work as a physician, I struggle with nearly everything except patient interaction. I am stressed by the computer systems, billing requirements, the challenges of accessing resources my patients need, and more. I don't pretend otherwise. That way, when I tell you that I relished seeing a patient who arrived with two police escorts after a prior physician refused to see that patient, who had threatened to kill him, you won't be so incredulous as to tune out the discussion that follows about why that encounter and the relationship that ensued were particularly rewarding.

Book Organization

The chapters are organized around topics that I found essential to my own development as a healer. The book begins with a description of the task-driven, all-consuming, hierarchical culture of medicine that marginalizes the patient and values—despite the rhetoric—only technical competence. Doctors learn to do stuff *to* people rather than *with* them, with few opportunities to see how it could be any other way. Chapter 1, titled "Physician or Technician?" illustrates the indoctrination process and how it molds the physician's mindset into that of a task completer rather than a thoughtful professional. It explores the countercurrents to becoming a healer, both in the training environment and in the larger society, that shape the people who go to medical school. Those countercurrents foster compartmentalization between the personal and professional, in addition to stymieing curiosity, self-trust, humility, and a capacity to engage.

Following the first chapter's exploration of the social forces that direct young adults, particularly those who enter medicine, to disengage and lose their curiosity, the second chapter, "Healing Interactions," begins with a discussion of the characteristics of a healer. A unifying theme is that healers exhibit an openness across their personal and professional relationships, combined with a high degree of self-awareness—often at odds with the prevailing culture. Hence, subsequent chapters explore the process of developing personally as well as professionally into a healer, especially during the formative years of becoming a physician, despite living and learning in an environment that frequently stifles that process.

Chapter 3, "Your Personal Journey," considers the personal growth entailed in becoming a healer. How do you take honest stock of where you are developmentally? Are you able to trust others, as reflected in being open with them about what you regard as your vulnerabilities? Do you trust in your own basic goodness? When things don't work out as you wanted, can you accept that you're not in control? Once, after I had my first panic attack in college, I commented to Simon that I didn't think I could turn to friends if I was having a panic attack as I feared they would think less of me. To which he replied, "Then what are friends for?" Learning to be vulnerable and trustworthy—which is to say nonjudgmental—immeasurably increases your value to your patients, particularly when they are suffering. You become someone who can be fully present for them and who is safe.

After having established the basic premises—that healers exhibit a set of personal qualities, that acquiring them is a personal journey, and that it requires overcoming countercurrents—three subsequent chapters explore the paths to "Overcoming Judgmentalism" (chapter 4), "Engaging with Boundary Clarity" (chapter 5), and "Caring" (chapter 6). The proposition of the first is that when we judge others we presume to know why they are behaving as they are, which shuts down curiosity. If you think you know why some of your patients don't take their medications—for instance, that they aren't taking your medical advice seriously—you have little motivation to explore what's really going on. The second describes how open and full engagement with boundary clarity is the foundation of any healing relationship, inside or outside of the practice of medicine. The terms *engagement* and *boundary clarity* are explored in depth, with an emphasis on examining what the terms mean and how they enable healing interactions. The chapter on caring also begins with a discussion of definitions, this time comparing the terms *caring* and *empathy*, which are often used interchangeably but warrant distinction. When you unselfishly care for someone, you'll take whatever actions you conclude will help them. To empathize has more to do with what one feels than how one acts. While empathy is widely assumed to increase caring behavior, that notion is challenged. However one defines the terms, what ultimately matters is not what you feel inside but what actions you take to elicit and address your patients' needs.

Eliciting and addressing patients' needs is the focus of chapter 7, "Making Medical Decisions." Unfortunately, medical training focuses too narrowly on diagnosing and treating disease. Care plans often look good on paper but fail because they don't take into account the circumstances or priorities of individual patients. This chapter introduces a practical framework for incorporating patients' life context and preferences into care planning without adding to the length of the clinical encounter. It applies concepts introduced in the prior three chapters, particularly the importance of replacing judgmentalism with curiosity so that you ask the right questions rather than make assumptions about patients' motivations and behaviors.

Chapter 8, "Healers Are Realists," explores how idealists become disillusioned in the face of messy reality, whereas realists work within it. There are various definitions of idealism, and I'm referring to this one: *the practice of forming or pursuing ideals, especially unrealistically.* The unrealistic part is often what idealists think they can accomplish, imagining they can swoop in and save the day. When the world doesn't respond as expected, disillusionment and then burnout set in. We hear people say things like, "I used to be so idealistic," with a rueful look of disappointment. Yet if idealism has its roots in unrealistic expectations, is it any surprise that it goes away? Disillusionment is often born of arrogance about what we thought we could accomplish.

In contrast, healers live in the real world, doing good work in harmony with their own lives. Chapter 8 introduces three physicians who are both pragmatists and healers, each in different ways.

Chapter 9, "Physician or Technician? (Revisited)," considers the problem addressed in chapter 1—why many physicians fall into a routine that is inattentive to patients' individual preferences and needs—from a different vantage point. Whereas the first chapter explores how the training experience constricts their capacity to relate to patients as individuals whose complicated lives complicate their health care, chapter 9 acknowledges that it's not always the physician who is the problem: In some practice environments, physicians are expected to see patients so fast that even if they engage, there's just no time to do more than order routine tests and institute care plans that look right on paper but may be ill-suited for any number of reasons that go unidentified or ignored. Physicians who find themselves in a situation in which they can't provide what they consider to be good care may ask themselves: Is this consistent with my principles? If the answer is no, it's time to make a change.

Chapter 10, "Healing as an Organizing Principle," explores what it means to approach every interaction as a healer, in a country that lately showcases meanness and bullying at the highest levels. Simon quotes the ethicist William F. May, who described the fully actualized physician as one who "eats to heal, drives to heal, reads to heal, comforts to heal, rebukes to heal, and rests to heal." Many might regard this way of life as exhausting and unrealistic. But they miss the point. What's exhausting is the inauthenticity and guardedness that characterize so many other ways of interacting. Healers let go of pretensions and posturing, which is liberating—and empowering. In a world with brutes, healers are resilient. As they know where they stand, they are not easily knocked off balance. Absent inflated egos, they are less prone to blindness born of self-deception. And, because their generosity does not go unnoticed, they accumulate friends in unexpected places who look out for them.

Unlike my previous book, *Listening for What Matters*, which is grounded in empirical research on interactions between patients and professionals who care for them, this one is based on what I've learned from a wise mentor and gained from experience. My conversations with Simon were almost always driven by questions I asked him, often about myself, as I wondered why I might be feeling or reacting to particular situations in particular ways during my training, or how I might better respond to something I encountered. Simon often responded by asking me what I thought and then guiding me to my own answers. The questions at the end of each chapter reflect these discussions.

I hope that as a reader you will find relevance to your life from much of what you come across in these pages, and that it will challenge you to grow personally as a healer such that your interactions with those who may be struggling or in pain—whether they are patients or not—are more comforting for them and fulfilling for you.

ONE

Physician or Technician?

A technician can be defined as one who knows every aspect of his job except its ultimate purpose and social consequences.

SIR RICHARD LIVINGSTON (ATTRIB.)

W HEN I was a first-year resident—an intern—I was struck by the uncomplaining endurance of my peers. We only spent about 15 percent of our time with patients; most of what we did was write orders and notes, stand in the hallway on rounds listening to or giving lengthy clinical presentations, and answer pages for an endless litany of requests from hospital staff requiring more orders and more notes. There's nothing odd about any of this—many jobs consist of mundane work—except that we did it for up to 110 hours a week during some months, and, when on call, for 36 or more hours at a time (current rules limit work stints to 80 hours a week and 28-hour shifts). Another strange thing was how infrequently people questioned the logic of what we were going through. In fact, there was a certain pride and gallows humor, with jokes like "the problem with every-other-night call is that you miss half the cases!"

Residents gave it their all, remaining remarkably conscientious even without sleep. One senior pediatric resident who supervised me looked for things to do well beyond what the patient came in for. During nights, I would try to finagle a way to get at least an hour of rest before a long "post-call day" that might not end until seven or eight o'clock. But that was rarely an option with Dr. Ivory, who drove her interns as hard as she drove herself. Nothing was back-burnered. Whether a child was admitted with an asthma attack or a concussion, she'd want a full review of the vaccination history before morning rounds, to see if the immunizations were up to date. That could require running down to the medical records department to locate the file (this was before the advent of the electronic medical record) as more patients flowed into the emergency department. She also requested I order lots of tests to look for rare conditions, and then follow up on the results right away. I found that if I did everything she wanted, she'd look at me approvingly, which I craved.

This perfectionist tendency is cultivated in medical school, where tests, typically multiple-choice, focus on minutiae, and where the attending physician might ask you anything about your patient's medical history, lab values, and so on. On the surface, such an exacting standard seems good for patient care. After all, who doesn't want a doctor who is full of facts? And doesn't hierarchy and a boot-camp environment foster exactitude, endurance, and discipline? It does. But the problem with obsessive behavior is that it represents a loss of perspective that comes with a price. Sure, if you keep checking whether your stove is on or your garage door is open, you might conceivably find one day that it is, but at what opportunity cost? What's left out of patient care as a result of such behavior?

What's left out is the individuality of the patient. We did things *to* people without finding out what challenges they were facing and what they most needed from us. Medical students and residents are immersed in a task-driven culture that objectifies the patients we are supposed to care about. At work I'd make long lists and then feel satisfied as each item got checked off, particularly on post-call days when "tucking all the patients in," as we called it, was the only way to get out— like parents who, after putting their children to bed, could finally rest. The first priority every morning was to discharge patients so their beds could be filled with new ones. A delay occurred if we had to meet with their families to discuss, for instance, whether they could return home or needed to go to a nursing home. One of the disincentives to spending time with patients was that doing so cut into time for completing tasks. Task completion drove us and was the measure of our success.

Doctors Don't Start Out This Way

How did such a state of affairs come to pass? First, it's important to acknowledge that practicing medicine really does require following a lot of steps. When patients are admitted to the hospital, the doctor's orders specify everything that happens, including what they will eat ("diabetic diet"), their activity level ("up in chair"), how often they'll be awakened at night ("vitals"), and what will happen if they stop breathing ("code status"). This all keeps staff busy. And when the various scans and blood work come back, the resident has to piece it all together to figure out what to do next. While challenging at first, it soon becomes routine. I remember the first time I admitted 12 patients during the night—the maximum allowed per call shift—with two interns under my supervision, and experienced the satisfaction of knowing that I knew what I was doing. I imagine it's similar to the pilot in training who gets to a point where they realize they're not likely to crash the plane, even in bad weather. Physician and pilot have, respectively, achieved competence.

However, a plane is an object, and a patient is a person. Philosopher and theologian Martin Buber distinguished between two ways of experiencing the world: as "I-It" or as "I-Thou," with the former referring to the manner in which we relate to people as if they were objects and the latter as how we should strive to relate to them as people. Unfortunately, we are prone to relate to others as objects once they have labels. Hence, "It" refers to all that we place into categories, including chairs, tables, and, yes, patients. Relating to a person as a "patient" is an "I-It" relationship when they are thought of as predominantly belonging to that category. Sometimes doctors subcategorize, and patients become "leukemics" or "diabetics," and so forth. Residency is almost perfectly designed to reinforce the "I-It" nature of the doctor-patient relationship when the latter becomes the object of a set of tasks.

How do we come to objectify other people, to relate to them as an "It" rather than a "Thou"? I don't think we start off that way. Our first interaction with another person is typically at our mother's breast. Within minutes of birth we enter into a reciprocal relationship where we cry for milk, and the more milk we consume, the more is produced. By six weeks of age we are making eye contact with our mother during breast feeding, and throughout the months that follow this relationship is paramount. The subsequent connections that we make, typically with another parent and/or sibling(s), are also highly engaged.

As infants we are so dependent on others for everything that we don't initially differentiate self from other. Such knowledge comes mostly through the experience of frustration—of not getting what we want when we want it, and hence realizing that what other people do is not under our control. Whereas we can put our hand in our mouth anytime we want, we can't make someone else put food in our mouth—we need to convince them to do that for us. We soon learn that the hand that feeds us belongs to someone else.

Hence boundary clarity, which may be defined as the capacity to differentiate that which is us from that which is not us, evolves as we adapt to life outside the womb. In the years that follow, we explore the world around us driven by insatiable curiosity. This is not just a human phenomenon. Kittens are famously curious, and their moms swat them away when they are about to try something foolhardy. Human parents do that too. I recall watching my daughter as a toddler put an extension cord in her mouth while observing me with a mischievous look on her face as I ran toward her to snatch it away. She did it repeatedly as a form of play that, while frustrating for me, taught her how to influence my behavior. As she got older, she became curious about nearly everything.

The point is that children, from early infancy, are eager to learn about the world and people around them. They soon acquire the basics: how to engage with key figures in their lives, an awareness of boundaries, and, after acquiring speech, the value of asking questions. So, what happens? How do we go from such a promising start to the gradual adoption of "I-It" and an uninquisitive acceptance of the status quo?

The disengaging process also starts early, with our parents signaling us to stay out of other people's business and not to talk with strangers for our safety (when, in fact, children are more likely to be victims of sexual or physical violence from people they know well). As a result, we develop an "us-them" mentality about the world, where the nuclear family is "us" and most of the world is "them." Just as our inclination to engage with anyone and everyone as a toddler is discouraged, so too is constant questioning. A problem with curiosity is that it can pose a threat to social conventions that maintain order through control and hierarchy. It's hard to explain many of those conventions to a logical, inquisitive mind. I recall my daughter as a preschooler questioning the rationale for table manners, conventions related to nudity in public, and how she could be sure we existed. Answering any one of these requires considerable thought, particularly with the added challenge of communicating with a person whose vocabulary and life experience are quite limited. Add to that the sheer volume of inquiries, which can wear parents down to the point where they rebuke children for asking questions. An exasperated response, such as "Because I said so," discourages curiosity.

It also cuts off the opportunity for engagement. Author and pediatrician Alan Greene observed that when his children asked, "Why is the sky blue?" they weren't just looking for information. In fact, concisely answering the question got a cold stare. What they wanted was an interaction, with give-and-take. A brief conversation about the different colors in the sky or the sun and the planets delighted them even if it didn't get around to addressing the question. I'd also add that returning to the original question is respectful, and looking for the answer together can be another shared activity.

Hence, curiosity and interpersonal engagement are intertwined in childhood, and shutting one down also shuts down the other. Schools, unfortunately, often suppress both with their emphasis on rewarding answers based on passive learning. It was sad to see, but I do recall that my daughter's curiosity diminished substantially as she entered high school, probably related to some poor but time-consuming course material. A required physics class began with instruction on how to predict the direction of an electromagnetic field as current flows through a wire, without any background on what an electromagnetic field is. She had to memorize a mnemonic involving pointing the thumb of her right hand up and making a fist. That was sufficient to pass the test.

Such abysmal course design is a turn-off for an inquisitive mind, yet still seems to be common even at top-ranked schools.

Similarly, premedical and medical school education can extinguish curiosity—and socioemotional development—by essentially holding the mind hostage. I learned early on that if I wanted to become a doctor, it was going to require intensively focusing on what I was told to do, and that it would entail years of preparing for high-stakes exams written by people who had immense power over how I spent my waking hours. If the writers of those tests are wise in their judgment of what future doctors need to know, then the system works. But if 30 percent, or 40 percent—or perhaps more than half—of the material is not relevant, then there is a massive opportunity cost. What are the costs of keeping students mentally exhausted by memorizing voluminous material they'll soon forget while they sacrifice acquiring other skills, both interpersonal and intellectual—including inquisitiveness? And, is this an unavoidable consequence of intensive training, or some form of social control?

In my first-year medical school immunology class I got slapped down early on when I questioned what we were taught. Although I wasn't a science major, I did take a year off between college and medical school to work in a molecular immunology laboratory with a pioneering team. A year later, when I discovered that the immunology instructor was teaching outdated material, I was savvy enough to know that I needed to broach the problem diplomatically. During a lab break, when I had a chance to discuss it out of earshot of others so as not to embarrass him, I showed him studies that were more current. I was careful to sound friendly and casual when I asked him what he thought of these newer findings, but it still didn't go well. What I heard was a variant of "Don't try to teach me immunology, you little pipsqueak." I recall thinking, as I went back to my lab bench and microscope, that I wasn't going to question anything else in medical school, and I didn't.

It's been said that "every system is perfectly designed to get the results it gets," and that's evident for the pipeline that produces doctors. Those students who are perfectly designed to gobble up information, rapidly learn new tasks, and not ask out-of-the box questions seem to flow smoothly along. The system is made for them. Those who can't fit the mold get stuck at some point, unable to pass. A middle group muddle through, but their slowness doesn't go unnoticed. I fit it into that third category. During residency, I was often asked, "Why are you still here?" on post-call days, as it took me longer to finish my work than most others who had already left to go home and sleep. An attending once observed that "if you were married, you wouldn't stay so late," as if I had nothing better to do than stumble around exhausted after 36 hours trying to finish up my work. Appearing efficient is what counted, perhaps even if it meant cutting corners, like spending less time than needed with a family or patient who needed to talk. The pressure was for conformity.

The Task-Driven Life

The go-go pace of internship seemed to suit a lot of my peers better than it suited me. This was in part because most were faster at learning how to do things than I. On morning rounds, the resident or attending would rattle off orders without enough information for me to follow what it was I was supposed to do. I'd jot down key words I'd heard and then later show them to another doctor to see if they could decipher what I was being told. My sense that I was not up to par was confirmed one afternoon, mid-internship, when my senior resident said, sternly, that I was "not performing at the level expected at this stage." I recall hearing this at least two or three times that year. During the first nine to ten months of residency, I often looked around and wondered if I could think of anyone who might be as slow and confused as I.

The residents who seemed so efficient and smart also hung out together, bar hopping on nights off. In medical school, and even as premeds, they were the cliques who knew how to work hard and party hard. In organic chemistry in college I recall students who exhibited a remarkable capacity to sit in lecture for hours every day filling up notebooks with neatly written, detailed mechanisms, followed by long lab sessions, followed by a high-stakes exam at the end of the week. Weekends were for catching up on sleep, followed by partying, and then back into the cycle early Monday mornings.

An important difference between me and most of my peers was my learning disability. It was something I couldn't run away from. I was aware that while others knew what was going on in class, I was lost. To survive I had to find new ways to learn on my own. I could not go out partying when I needed to keep my mind in top form at all times so that I could focus on my studies. I've often wondered how actors and rock stars are so productive while drinking so much and getting high. How do they even remember their lines on stage when they're intoxicated or stoned? Medical school prompted the same wonderment at my peers' cognitive abilities under self-imposed duress.

Others who pursue professional training soon after college, such as most law students, have similar lives, what some call a prolonged adolescence. But there is a difference, which is the destination. The destination for future physicians is not a corporate office or a firm. It is at the bedside of a woman, man, or child who is frail, frightened, in pain, nearly naked in a hospital gown, or in some other way vulnerable and exposed—a person with fears and needs that twenty-somethings who are generally healthy, ambitious, task-oriented, and prone to escapism do not often contemplate.

It's not that all medical school students have led rosy lives and are unfamiliar with struggle and suffering; it's that personal struggles are concealed and inner turmoil suppressed. When I was training, it seemed as if nobody had any problems—except when awful things happened, such as when a resident I occasionally took call with committed suicide about a week before completing the program. People kept their struggles to themselves, and that appeared to suit the administration just fine. While there was probably a counseling service one could seek out, I don't recall anyone telling us about it.

At the medical school where Simon taught for over 30 years, he maintained an open door policy—literally—in order to give students a place to confide their struggles. Over the years he heard countless stories about child abuse, spousal abuse, substance abuse, depression, posttraumatic stress disorder (PTSD), and other sources of suffering among a group of young people who looked on the surface like they had won life's lottery. Simon quoted Thoreau's dictum that "the mass of men lead lives of quiet desperation." He once commented that while he thought it was hyperbole the first time he heard it, he didn't think so anymore. Like their patients, many young physicians know despair. But the conventions of medical training do not facilitate coming to terms with emotions. Rather, trainees bottle up feelings and focus on projecting assuredness as they move from task to task and patient to patient. Emotionally stunted, they are inaccessible to their patients, as they are inaccessible to themselves.

I'm not implying that self-knowledge is a necessary prerequisite for a contented life or to be good at a job. It's just that it is if you are a physician. Surely, many who are not inclined toward self-examination are good neighbors, hard workers, and trustworthy to their family and friends alike. My dentist described his dad, an immigrant from Greece, that way, saying, "He was still parking cars at Wrigley Field for Cubs games when he was 85 years old, and sharp as a tack. He never reflected much about himself, as far as I could see, but we always knew we could count on him."

Simon observed that, in this respect, Socrates was wrong when he famously said, "The unexamined life is not worth living." But the adage does apply to physicians, who must examine themselves and the lives they live because of the work they do and the socialization pressures of medical training. Otherwise they will adopt disengaged behaviors and rigid ways of thinking. After mastering book learning and multiple-choice test taking, they enter the clinical years of their training applying the same skills of compulsively completing assigned tasks. They mimic what they observe. Hence, if their professors talk down to them, they adopt similar ways of relating to more junior trainees and to patients. Because they expect perfection of themselves, they avoid delving too deeply into the struggles their patients are facing for fear they won't know what to do with what they hear. When their patients are unappreciative or even oppositional, they take it personally, lacking the boundary clarity to recognize this isn't about them.

Unprepared, developmentally, for the doctor-patient relationship in its real life complexity, they retreat. In place of a fulfilling career with meaningful relationships with patients is a job like any other job, with paperwork, procedures, and a way of relating that has been described as emotional labor. *Emotional labor* is a term used in the service industry when, for instance, flight attendants must mask emotions they feel and portray emotions they don't feel. It's fake relating to meet the expectations of the customer and employer.

Not everyone enters medicine looking for fulfillment through healing relationships with patients. Some are attracted to the high earning potential, the status, or simply job security. But even among the materially minded, many desire to have a positive impact. I remember that my classmates who sought careers in surgery said that for them, the reward would be "going in there and fixing the problem." Inpatient medicine, in contrast, with its endless rounds and stream of patients with progressive, chronic conditions cycling in and out of the hospital, struck them as hopelessly ungratifying. Outpatient medicine, with its "worried well," would be a waste of time or more of the same. I recall thinking that it was difficult to argue with them.

Only years later have I come to appreciate the fallacy. First, surgery doesn't necessarily fix things. What it does is slice someone open, with the potential to do irreversible harm. Tens of thousands of people have had their backs or their prostates operated on with no gain, or with devastating consequences. Some have benefited greatly. So, the premise that a career in surgery will spare the physician the messy uncertainties of trying to help people whose bodies are still largely a mystery to the medical profession is false. It reflects a desire to cling to an expectation of perfection that characterizes many who want to become doctors and who are able to make it into and through medical school.

Second, caring for patients with chronic conditions, or simply the vagaries of old age, isn't just about ordering lab tests, CT scans, and pills while watching them slowly recede toward death. It's about helping people cope with and adapt to what's happening to their bodies as they live their lives. But to serve patients in that way requires emotional and cognitive capabilities that aren't discussed in medical school and are rarely modeled by faculty. With that piece missing, the perception of those heading into surgery that medicine is a Sisyphean task isn't far off the mark. Internal medicine and primary care really are demoralizing if you think of patients as walking checklists of tasks to complete each time you see them.

What I've observed is that surgeons run from human engagement but can't hide from it, whereas medicine doctors are drawn to it but are unprepared for what comes their way. These are generalizations, of course, that apply to many but certainly not to all. Among all types of physicians are those who do in fact openly and fully engage. To those who wonder where they fall, I pose the following question: Do you find interactions with your patients nourishing, and leading over time to a sense of attachment? That's what engagement feels like. Those who answer "yes" are fortunate to have a personally and professionally rewarding career, and their patients—whether they appreciate it or not—are cared for by a healer. While healers appreciate being appreciated, it's not what makes their work fulfilling, and its absence doesn't diminish their sense of fulfillment.

The problem is that too few physicians find patient interactions nourishing, likely because they have been unable to retain the curiosity and openness to engage that they exhibited in their early lives. As discussed, there are many pressures to become less open and accessible to others, and to prioritize conforming over questioning as we grow up. The consequences for physicians and their patients are mutually adverse. Many physicians slog on, unfulfilled in their work, in the same manner that many people accommodate unfulfilling marriages. The connections are not there. Patients may or may not know what they're missing. They often expect surprisingly little from their doctors other than technical competence and amicability. But, unfortunately, this often means settling for less than they need. There is relatively little in medicine that is so cut and dried that a lack of engagement isn't consequential.

"You Come by It Honestly"

It is a paradox that we are prone to pass on to the next generation the destructive behaviors of those who hurt us. One study showed that pediatricians who were spanked by their parents were more likely to endorse spanking, despite seeing the research evidence that it teaches kids that violence solves problems and doesn't lead to better behavior. As adults, we often repackage our trauma and inflict it on others in a modified form. It can be quite subtle. In my early 20s and 30s I could put others down when I felt insecure to show that I knew more than they did. Simon—who knew my mom well—would say, "You come by it honestly."

Many people, if not most, experience enough micro-trauma to hold others at a distance. The commonality that I've observed frequently in relationships characterized by power imbalances—employer/employee, teacher/student, and parent/child—is capricious heavy-handedness. The parent or teacher or employer seems caring and supportive, leading the child, student, or employee to open up, to begin to relax and trust, and then, bam! They unexpectedly cut them down to size. Such impulses are born out of insecurity expressed as showing who's in charge.

Simon guided me through reframing: A few years into my job as the director of a residency training program, when I was just a few years older than the physicians I supervised, I got irritated by a resident who used to e-mail me with the salutation "Hey, Saul . . ." rather than the more customary "Dear Dr. Weiner . . ." or "Dear Saul . . ." I felt I was not being respected. When I asked Simon what he thought I should do, he replied, "What's disrespectful about how she's addressing you? It's informal and probably means she's comfortable with you. However, I do think you should let her know that while it's fine for her to address you that way, you want to be sure she's aware to be cautious about such informality with future employers." Rather than chiding her, he guided me to educate her in a manner that was no longer about me. When I talked with her, she seemed appreciative and relaxed. Had I reprimanded her, I could have undermined our relationship. I would have passed on that same capricious heavy-handedness.

Parents have the biggest impact because they create the world we inhabit in our early, most impressionable, years, at a time when we have no points of reference. They also shape how we behave years later when we have some power. I recall the terror I would feel when I said something my mother perceived as "being fresh" and her face would go dark with rage. By the time I realized what I had done, it was too late. Yet her reaction indicated she thought I was intentionally provoking her. Without the mentorship I got from Simon, I may have repeated the same behavior.

Similarly, I've learned that my physician colleagues who complain about patients who "never listen," or who "are never satisfied no matter what I do" have a worldview that they likely "came by honestly." They take things personally that have nothing to do with them. Preoccupied with their own emotional response, they react to angry patients with defensiveness rather than openness to understanding what they are observing. They do their best to conceal their feelings, of course, and act as if they are above the fray, which can seem patronizing. Instead, they could be asking what is going on when a patient's behavior seems irrational or counterproductive: Why are patient and doctor so not on the same page? Why might the patient seem so chronically dissatisfied, and what's the therapeutic response? If the doctor is preoccupied with how they are treated—if, in other words, it's about them and not the patient—such questions are likely overlooked. Overlooking them not only compromises patient care but diminishes both parties. The individuality of the patient has not been acknowledged, and the physician is living in self-imposed solitary confinement, having cut themselves off from meaningful interaction. Medicine gets dull fast when it's just about knowing what pills to prescribe or tests to order. The richness comes from real human connection.

To engage, you must regard your patient as an equal, despite differences in your medical knowledge or overall education. It may help to remember, for instance, that a homeless man or woman living on the streets in the dead of winter has survival skills you'd sorely need were you to land in their situation. An openness to engage comes out of an appreciation for the universality of the human experience and an understanding that differences are due to chance. If you can acknowledge that we all sometimes smell bad, look bad, and end up in really embarrassing situations, it's easy to be responsive to a patient's needs, as they cease to be "other." After doing a foot exam you might offer to put a sock back on as a patient struggles to bend over, or after completing a rectal exam, you could ask the patient if they would like you to wipe the sticky gel from their behind rather than just handing them tissue paper to do it themselves.

Unexpected small gestures such as these can have a lasting effect. When I was sixteen, I stayed with Simon for a week at his home in Washington, DC. As I already aspired to be a physician, he invited me to the medical school to sit in on a class he taught. He woke me by gently knocking on the door at 6:00 a.m. and entering with a glass of freshly squeezed orange juice on a tray. No one had ever done anything like that for me, and it seemed a bit odd. However, over time I came to appreciate that such graciousness is characteristic of how he relates to everyone, regardless of their status, education, or responsibilities relative to his.

How we are treated greatly shapes how we treat others. Many of us have little experience with unconditional caring and respect. Patients come to expect and accept a low bar for how they're treated by their doctors because they don't know anything different. They acquiesce to physicians who do most of the talking and rarely ask questions, because what other options do they have? Nevertheless, they want to believe their doctor is great, as reflected in national patient satisfaction data that show how few doctors get less than a four- or five-star rating. Such expectations extend beyond health care: Students look up to teachers who spoon-feed them information and don't like to be challenged, both because it feels familiar and because they don't know what they are missing. And we all too often pick life partners ignoring—or perhaps embracing—the familiar feeling of not being treated well. Our expectations are set by the formative relationships we have when we are young, starting with our parents. And for many the bar stays low. That is unless we have the good fortune to have someone in our lives who shows us what a high bar looks like.

Unfortunately, medical school faculty who teach physician-patient communication rarely model open and full engagement. Instead, students are taught to navigate the doctor-patient relationship through practiced behaviors. They take classes on topics such as "giving bad news" and "communicating empathy." While well intentioned, the training nevertheless orients them to "do something" to people, rather than to make a genuine human connection. They become proficient technicians rather than healing professionals.

Questions for Reflection and Discussion

1. When you reflect on how you practice medicine, do you think you are functioning mainly as a technician, or is your decision making taking into account particulars of each patient's unique situation and preferences? If the latter, what are some examples?

2. When you are with a patient who has, say, poorly controlled diabetes, how far do you think you should go toward understanding what is going on? Are you likely just to ask if they are taking their current medications correctly and then adjust them as needed? Or are you the doctor who figures out that their vision has been failing so they can't read the insulin syringe reliably, they've become fearful of injecting themselves regularly, and that what they really need now is both an ophthamology referral and prefilled syringes?

3. If you're the second kind of doctor in the example above who gets to the bottom of things going on in your patients' lives that affect their care, do you find this detective work exasperating, rewarding, or something else? Do you think it's your job, or are you going beyond what's expected of a physician practicing competently?

4. How has your training enhanced or impeded your functioning at a level above that of a technician who provides technically competent care that looks correct if you examine the chart, but is probably not ideal if you know what's going on with the patient?

[TWO]

Healing Interactions

The secret of the care of the patient is in caring for the patient.

FRANCIS W. PEABODY, MD

WE'VE PROBABLY all had brief interactions, sometimes with strangers, that leave us feeling better than we felt a few minutes earlier. We may remember those moments as a "breath of fresh air." Physician and author Rachel Naomi Remen, who has written and talked about living with Crohn's disease, describes just such an encounter with a nurse that may have saved her life. It was a particularly dark period for her, in the 1960s, when as a young physician in her late 20s she had major surgery at the hospital where she also worked. The surgery involved removal of a large section of her intestine and placement of an ostomy bag. At the time it was considered high risk and experimental. During the long recovery period, colleagues and friends came by to cheer her up. Meanwhile, she was descending into a deep depression, unable to imagine her life as a young woman with a bag containing fecal material extruding from her abdomen. She began secretly hoarding the sedatives placed at her bedside each evening, with plans to take them all at once after she left the hospital to end her life. She'd decided that she didn't want to do it while she was still there, as she thought it would humiliate the doctors and nurses caring for her.

A chance visit by an ostomy nurse, however, changed everything. Up to that moment, Remen had grown accustomed to being treated in a way that made her feel like a medical specimen. Staff were courteous, but their behaviors betrayed squeamishness. They came to change her ostomy bag extensively gowned. They seemed efficient and courteous, but distant. The nurse who came in this time was different. It was a weekend evening, and she was dressed fashionably, on her way out to a social event. Remen wasn't in her usual hospital garb either, as she was wearing a colorful outfit her friends had gotten to lift her spirits. This was a setup for a demoralizing encounter: her caretaker living in a world of normalcy and fun, while she, all alone and stuck in the hospital, could only dress the part. But the nurse didn't see things that way. She conversed as one young woman to another, chatting unselfconsciously about their clothing, things to do in town and so forth, as might two friends chatting at a café. Remen almost forgot her situation.

She also noticed that while the nurse was meticulous at washing her hands so as to avoid infecting the healing wound, she didn't bother putting on protective garb. In reality, there was no need to do so, as Remen wasn't infectious. The others may have been acting out of fear, not of infection but of physical contact. This nurse, in contrast, was simply providing a helping hand while having a pleasant time. She was both warmly informal and highly professional. Remen said she never saw that nurse again, but the 15 minutes together literally saved her life. As the woman left, Remen was able for the first time since her surgery to see a place for herself in the world. Someone had regarded the ostomy as inconsequential, simply a practical matter rather than what defines a person. Hope returned and the desire to die receded.

When we are feeling insecure and unsure of ourselves, we are particularly sensitive to how others regard us. It wasn't the ostomy that had Remen so depressed. It was how people responded to her in her new state. It took just one person who related to her as normal to change everything. Not objectifying her patient also enabled the nurse to enjoy a human interaction. She related to Remen rather than to Remen's wound. She saw a young woman like herself, so that's how she related to her. She wasn't caught up in the fear and "otherness" that infected the rest of the team. As a result, she got to be herself.

Healing interactions are mutually nourishing, because they are based on real human connection. They occur not only in hospitals and clinics but at work, at the gym, or on a bus. A woman I worked with got stuck in an elevator with someone more senior in the organization who tended to be aloof and reserved. This individual, however, suffering from claustrophobia and needing reassurance, let his guard down. Unexpectedly, it was just two people supporting each other in a situation where their status outside the elevator no longer mattered. They were literally and figuratively on the same level. They maintained a friendly rapport after that experience.

Frightening or isolating situations create a heightened need for emotional support, which opens individuals to meaningful human interaction, including those who are typically guarded. Even if temporarily, they also level the playing field. It's said that there is no racism on the battlefield. When your life is on the line, all you care about is that your fellow soldiers have your back, not the color of their skin. The conditions of life in combat obliterate social constructs that stratify people under normal circumstances.

In the medical encounter, the physician is generally the impediment to such meaningful interaction, which I've referred to as *engagement*. Patients are typically ready or even hungry to engage. They are the ones feeling trapped, on a battlefield of sorts, or simply in need of human connection at a time when they feel vulnerable. Meanwhile, their doctor is having just another busy day at work. The usual justification for not engaging is that there isn't enough time. But the question is whether they would interact differently if they had all the time in the world. And, more fundamentally, is an openness to fully engage even time-dependent? Or, rather, is it simply a way of relating to people?

An openness to engage is a show of respect. It means you consider the person worthy of your full attention. You are curious about what they have to say because you want to understand where they're coming from. You presume that however puzzling their behavior may seem, they have their reasons. You regard them as an equal at a fundamental level, neither expecting that you know what's right for them, nor that you should do whatever they want.

According them your full attention, however, is not the same as according them unlimited attention. Positive engagement must be circumscribed by boundaries. Boundaries demarcate who we are both in the literal sense (that is, our skin) and in terms of our values, preferences, and obligations. Just as physicians should respect patients' boundaries, they should maintain their own. For doctors, staying on schedule so as not to keep other patients waiting is an obligation. If you're going to run over the allotted time with a patient, it should be because you have consciously decided it's the right thing to do, under the circumstances, not because the patient "won't let you go." I've found that physicians are often uncomfortable telling patients it's time to end visits, so that they frequently run over. Such behavior reflects a lack of boundary clarity.

One problem with lacking boundary clarity is that physicians are reluctant to engage in the first place because they fear that if they "open Pandora's box" they won't be able to close it. When I think a patient may need more time than I have, I'll mention at the start of the visit that "Unfortunately, the bean counters only gave you twenty minutes of my time today, but if it's helpful to you, we can schedule another visit or make other arrangements to talk further if we run out of time." I regard such fair notice as a courtesy to the patient so they can prioritize, and a way to keep myself on track. It also sends a message not to take my ending the visit personally. The point is that there are straightforward logistical workarounds to the common reasons physicians give for not engaging with their patients, including that they don't have time.

One indicator that a physician is engaging is that they "contextualize care." As described in the introduction, a plan of care is contextualized when it's adapted to a patient's individual needs and circumstances. If you're engaged, you won't ignore a comment like, "Boy, it's been tough since I lost my job" in a patient who may have stopped taking a medication as evidenced by a flare-up of their asthma symptoms. Instead, you'll ask what they mean. If they tell you that they can't afford the costly brand-name medication they're taking, you'll switch them to a less costly generic. In contrast, ignoring such a comment and simply adding more medication reflects inattention to context. It's what happens when physicians don't engage. As a result, one of the practical benefits of engaging with patients is that it enables better care. Physicians become curious about what is going on with the person in front of them. If a patient with previously well-controlled diabetes has a high glycosylated hemoglobin, they are bound to ask, "Ms. Jones, what happened?" rather than lecture her or simply add more medicine.

One of the most striking findings in our research on contextualization of care, as noted earlier, is that it doesn't lengthen visits. Physicians who take the time to figure out why a patient isn't doing well save an equal amount of time during the encounter avoiding pointless discussions about adding new therapies and treatments that are ineffectual. Hence, the reasons physicians don't engage are intrinsic to them, not to the constraints of the medical encounter. Either they don't know how to engage, or they don't want to, or some of both. Engaging with patients isn't going to happen if it's perceived as additional effort and work—if it's seen as yet "one more thing I'm supposed to do during a busy, draining day" rather than a refreshing way of relating to people.

I think the notion that interacting with patients is a task, rather than a way of being, is inadvertently reinforced when doctor-patient communication is taught in medical schools. Typically, in the first and second years, there is a "doctoring" course that teaches communication with patients, along with how to conduct a history and physical exam. There are a variety of instructional techniques, including small group discussions, interviews with simulated patients, observing faculty with real patients, role-playing, and videotaping. The classes or seminars generally share in common that they teach communication as a set of skills, often involving steps to carry out during a medical encounter. Trainees are taught to "build rapport," "demonstrate empathy," "engage in active listening," "project calmness," and so forth. Many communications skills curricula in medical school consist of tasks such as "opening the discussion" or "understanding the patient's perspective." Students are given specific directives, such as "allow the patient to complete his or her opening statement," and "be aware that ideas, feelings and values of the patient and doctor influence the relationship." You'll find many such directives in online syllabi and instructional publications.

The whole approach reminds me of learning to paint by numbers. I recall a communication class during my second year of medical school in which it was my turn to interview a standardized patient while the teacher graded me as my classmates sat around and watched. I tried to follow explicit instructions about when to lean forward, where to sit, and when to make eye contact. I had trouble keeping track of these tasks and lost quite a few points. It's no wonder that students' communication skills deteriorate as they progress through their training. Rather than be encouraged, whatever intuition they may have about how to relate to people is overridden instead by an approach that is formulaic.

I don't think that is the intent of those who design and teach communication classes. Rather, I believe it is to provide tools and strategies for enhancing the abilities that students bring with them. The classes are also attempting to address a legitimate need, particularly when preparing students for high-stakes conversations about difficult topics such as serious illness and death. While teaching helpful tips, however, these classes are ignoring the elephant in the room: namely, fear. On the one hand, in a capricious world where illness and misfortune can strike at any time, we all need each other. On the other, in the face of suffering, we are prone to retreat out of a sense of our own vulnerability. Falling back on a scripted set of tactics, beginning with "building rapport," is better than fleeing in the face of suffering, but it falls far short of what the situation requires. It is a form of hiding.

What is the difference between "building rapport" and attempting to engage? Superficially they may seem similar, but the differences are profound. Engaging is a personal expression of caring. "Building rapport" is a labor. I recall watching my attending physician on the oncology service attempt in vain to build rapport with a desperately unhappy woman whose husband had left her after she was diagnosed with cancer and hospitalized for a bone marrow transplant. She wanted to go home and die. The attending said, speaking in a soft voice, that he understood how bad she must feel and that he hoped she would consider the implications of leaving. He also said he'd like her to meet with a psychologist. She didn't stay. Something about his approach wasn't effective.

The incident came back to mind years later—along with an opportunity to think about a more effective approach—when I came across a similar case reported by the physician and philosopher Jodi Halpern in her book *From Detached Concern to Empathy: Humanizing Medical Practice*, about a 56-year-old woman with diabetes who had developed complications of renal failure, and peripheral vascular disease requiring bilateral above-the-knee amputations. The patient, whom Halpern refers to as "Ms. G," declined life-sustaining hemodialysis when her husband left her for another woman. Halpern recalls that, as she approached the patient's room in the hope of talking her out of it, friends standing outside said, "Ask her about her husband, that creep." When she met with Ms. G, she attempted to build rapport, beginning indirectly with, "Is there anything besides your body that is hurting you?" Ms. G replied, "My husband doesn't love me anymore. He told me that he's in love with someone else. He moved in with her while I was in the hospital. He said that with my amputations and other medical problems, he could never be attracted to me." Relating what had happened to her heightened the women's pain, which she suddenly directed at Halpern in rage, crying out, "Why the hell did you ask me to talk about this? . . . Don't ask me any more questions! Get out of here!" Halpern relates how, at a loss, she exited the woman's room and discussed the situation with several male supervising physicians who concluded that since the woman was mentally competent, they must respect her feelings. She was sedated and died shortly thereafter. For years Dr. Halpern says she has revisited this case, speaking about it and considering whether a different interaction could have had a better outcome.

What might a highly personal, heartfelt response have looked like at the point where Ms. G got angry and demanded her doctor leave? When I asked Simon, he was visibly upset that a woman would let a man run roughshod over her with such dire consequences, and replied, "I'd say: 'I'll leave, if you insist. But before I do, there's something I need to say, and even though it may sound harsh to you, if I understand you correctly, it's something you need to hear. I hear you saying that you want to die so that asshole who once professed to you his undying love and commitment can walk off with everything you own and give it to that women he's just moved in with! No! What you need is to get the nastiest divorce lawyer in town who'll take him for all he's worth for abandoning this poor, disabled woman—and I'll help you find that person! Don't reward the sonofabitch! Make him pay! And see how long his new girlfriend wants him around!' " Simon and I proposed this response in our essay "From Empathy to Caring: Defining the Ideal Approach to a Healing Relationship."

Such an approach to a patient's rage is unconventional. I hesitated to share it because it could be misunderstood as sanctioning aggressive and vulgar language with patients. But it exemplifies where rapport building and an engaged response diverge. It goes beyond caring for a patient to caring *about* them. Simon's objective in expressing his feelings is to convert the patient's grief and despair into anger, to mobilize and energize her to defend her dignity rather than surrender to an unfortunate situation. What distinguishes this as a professional response, despite its crudeness, is that the anger is directed at her passively allowing herself to be victimized, rather than at her husband. Simon's intentional use of offensively crude, vulgar language to convey his anger and to exhort a course of action is a caring response, based on a calculated assessment of the situation: That bold actions are needed since the patient's emotional situation is extremely dire and will soon lead to her death without such an intervention; that she is clearly capable of rage; and that she is not lacking for support in this cause, given that friends are advocating for her. That willingness to step outside of professional norms when it might save a life is a hallmark of engagement and exemplifies caring.

Remen's and Simon's examples illustrate radically different ways of relating, each suited to their situation, and reflect the personalities of the individuals and the exigencies of the moment. What they share in common is that they are coming from a person, not a persona.

Engaging with others is the shortest path to caring about them. When you care about someone, you become personally invested in their well-being. I noticed that happening to me as a junior resident when I met a man my age, in his late 20s, on the inpatient service for a flare-up of his sickle cell disease. I learned that Arthur had been admitted dozens of times with sickle cell pain crises, that he would "demand" specific narcotics, then leave against medical advice (AMA), and not follow up at his outpatient appointments. Many of his hospitalizations were serious enough that he required blood transfusions. As a result he developed hemochromatosis—iron overload—which damaged his organs, including his liver. He was advised to start deferoxamine intravenous therapy, a medication that helps remove the iron, but hadn't followed up with the referrals to hematology. Arthur was considered the worst kind of patient: demanding, unreliable, belligerent, and manipulative. I was warned that he was "drug seeking" and that I should "be on my guard."

It's odd, when you think about it, that doctors are frightened by patients. They feared that this slight 26-year-old with a profoundly disabling disease, who'd never finished high school, would push them around. And in a manner Arthur did so, at a small cost to their egos and at a huge cost to himself. One could say he was "messing with them." In an excruciatingly painful world in which he spent much of his time in the hospital with little or no say about what he ate or how he spent his day, keeping his doctors off-balance might have given him some small sense of control, however dysfunctional the dynamic. While they held him at arm's length, he took swings at them, pushing their backs against the wall. He was engaging negatively, and they weren't engaging at all. It occurred to me that if he could make them so uncomfortable, he was probably pretty bright.

What accounted for this dynamic? I suspect his doctors hadn't engaged with him because they didn't know how. They weren't open about what they were thinking, which he resented and exploited. He would say things like, "Are you saying you don't believe me when I tell you Demerol is the only pain killer that works for me?" and they would respond, "It's not that I don't believe you, it's that I think we should try something else . . ." and he'd tie them in pretzels as he pointed out that they had just contradicted themselves. A more candid response would have been to say that they didn't know him well enough to know if they could believe him, and that they weren't comfortable risking their medical license by writing a potentially unsafe prescription. They feared telling him what they were thinking, which he recognized as disrespectful, so he taunted them.

When I first met Arthur, stepping into his hospital room and introducing myself as the doctor who would be caring for him, I was surprised by his personality, given what I'd heard. He seemed relaxed, made eye contact, and although we didn't talk much, I noticed that he used language with agility. Working in an urban hospital on the South Side of Chicago I'd cared for many patients who were difficult to communicate with because their language skills were hampered by the environment in which they were raised. As someone with a learning disability who had benefited immensely from excellent schools, private tutoring, and parents who read to me as a small child, I was acutely aware that the difference between me and the impoverished men and women who struggled to express themselves was simply luck of circumstance. There but for the grace of God go I. I also appreciated that when I met a poor young man who was articulate and sharp despite a life of severe chronic illness and little education, I was in the presence of someone with high intelligence. As he and I started to talk, I thought, "this is someone I think I can connect with."

My initial approach with Arthur was to come by his room and show high interest in his health and health care before he was discharged. I carefully reviewed his medical records and wanted him to see that I'd made the effort, asking him about how his condition was affecting his life, what medications he was taking, and so forth. I saw it as a kind of audition, and I wanted to pass. The conversation was only about 10 minutes, but probably more than he was used to. I told him that I thought he needed to continue to use narcotics to control his pain but I believed he should switch from meperidine (Demerol) to morphine, since the former could cause seizures at such high levels and was likely more addictive because of its fast action and associated euphoria, which seemed to be leading to escalating dosages. As I anticipated, Arthur objected to switching to a different narcotic, saying that only Demerol worked to control his pain. I stood my ground, saying I would prescribe an equivalent dose, and explaining that "I am personally not comfortable keeping you on that medication, as I believe it is more likely to harm you, and I'm not prepared to take that risk." He told me he'd probably need to find another doctor. I responded that he could do that if he thought that was the right thing, but that I hoped that he would stick with me because I was looking forward to getting to know him and seeing if I could be helpful. My comment might have puzzled him, as the usual dynamic had been his pushing his doctors away and their being more than ready to see him look for care somewhere else. He grudgingly agreed to come to my outpatient clinic in a week.

Not surprisingly, he didn't show up. As soon as clinic was over I gave him a call. He seemed surprised but pleased to hear from me. He said he couldn't make it because he was watching over a couple of nieces and nephews, and I could hear kids playing in the background. We chatted about his family, and I asked him how he was getting along. He said he was doing okay. I told him I wanted him to see a specialist to get on a medication called hydroxyurea, which could reduce the frequency of his sickle cell crises. He agreed to do that, and I scheduled the consultation.

On the appointed day, I logged into the computer system and saw that he was a "no show." Again I called him, and this time he didn't have an excuse other than that he'd forgotten. I said, "Arthur, you're too smart to forget something this important. What's going on?" He told me that a friend of his had gotten shot and he was feeling awful about it. We discussed what had happened. He told me that he wasn't involved with gangs anymore but had been, despite his sickle cell disease. Now he was "an old man" and didn't get into trouble anymore. We laughed about that.

From then on he began showing for appointments with me, and finally followed up in hematology, where he was started on hydroxyurea, a daily pill that can decrease the rate of painful sickle cell crisis episodes. In addition, the hematologist started deferoxamine to try to remove some of the excessive iron that had accumulated in his body after years of blood transfusions. By the time I met Arthur, it had infiltrated his liver and heart, causing irreversible damage. We tried nevertheless in the hope that, given a chance, perhaps his body could heal itself. Deferoxamine requires a nightly eight-hour infusion using a pump—for a period of months in severe cases like his. That entailed arranging for a home nurse to visit and a social worker to coordinate his care. He accommodated these changes in his life.

Our interactions didn't always go smoothly. After we had a solid relationship that seemed personal and at times intimate, he started to demand that I switch him back to Demerol, saying he had no reason to see me if I wasn't going to treat him right. These outbursts were disconcerting and a bit hurtful, although I realized they were an indication that he was struggling. They reminded me of a child having a temper tantrum as a way of releasing pent-up feelings. Rather than saying "What the hell is wrong with you? We've been getting along great," I took each one at face value: "I'm sorry you're miserable. What's going on?" He'd see that I asked a lot of questions, was obviously concerned, but wasn't going to give him Demerol. The outbursts coincided with his growing appreciation that his hemochromatosis was severe and that while we could buy him some time, he was nearing the end of his life. This was something he figured out himself and first brought up with me. As I came to understand that his eruptions were a testament that he felt safe that I wouldn't abandon him, I took them as a sign of trust rather than as hurtful. Whenever I had the opportunity I shared with him my appreciation for his insight and intelligence, based on something he had just said or done. He would nod appreciatively but never looked surprised. I got the sense that he knew he was smart. On the other hand, he'd probably not often had this part of him acknowledged.

Arthur died one night from complications of the hemochromatosis on his heart, causing heart failure culminating in a fatal heart rhythm. A home nurse notified me, and I called his mother. I recall, a week later, pulling into the parking lot at the funeral parlor in Auburn Gresham, a neighborhood twenty minutes southwest of Hyde Park, where I worked. A lot of people were there, and everyone was dressed up. I was the only white person in sight. No one stared at me, although I felt self-conscious. When I stepped into the parlor, Arthur's mother spotted me and came over. I clasped her hand. A few minutes later one of the ushers said that Ms. Barnes (not her real name) would like for me to sit next to her. I felt awkward and undeserving of this request—but knew it was what I should do. I sat next to her during the service. There was an open casket, so I had a chance to see Arthur one last time.

For about a year after that I kept in touch with Ms. Barnes, calling her now and then to see how she was getting along. The tragedy of the story is that Arthur might have lived a long life had he started on deferoxamine years earlier. It was already well established at the time that early chelation therapy, as it's called, prevents iron buildup and organ damage, and our hospital was providing the service to other patients who received frequent transfusions. Arthur's medical record noted that he was "noncompliant" and therefore not a candidate for a medication that required nightly infusions and close monitoring. He certainly should have been.

The problem was that the doctors lacked the interpersonal competencies to care for Arthur. As noted, they were turned off by his behavior because they lacked boundary clarity and, perhaps as a result, were unwilling or unable to engage. When he gave them a hard time, they took it personally or assumed it was a fixed trait of his character. Reacting based on how one feels in response to a patient's behavior rather than on the responsibilities one accepts as their physician represents a lack of boundary clarity. Assuming their behavior is a personality characteristic rather than asking them what is going on represents a lack of engagement.

These clinician deficits can be lethal as well as common. Arthur was judged incapable of participating in care that he needed when he was perfectly able to. In fact, the doctors had the problem reversed: They were the ones incapable of giving him the care he needed. By "care" I'm not referring just to the medical services he should have received, that is, the medications to reduce his symptoms and treat the iron deposition. That's not "care"; that's technical know-how. To "care" is to "feel concern or interest; to look after and provide for the needs of." Because of his physicians' inability to care he wasn't able to benefit from their technical know-how.

I enjoy caring for patients labeled "difficult" for a couple of reasons. First, one can sometimes break the cycle of dysfunction between the patient and the health care system, leading to unexpected improvements in their health status. This is personally rewarding. If a patient is dying of cancer because every possible drug has failed, there isn't much one can do to save them. But if their health care is a mess because of conflicted relationships with their care team, there is the potential to make a difference. Second, I find "difficult" patients stimulating because their antagonism is an indication that there is an unresolved backstory. Why in the world is this person behaving in a way that is self-defeating? That's a challenge to explore.

Unfortunately, not all patients respond positively to an engaged, caring physician. Some are incapable of trust. Their past experiences, often dating back to early childhood, are so fraught with abusive or controlling interactions that they have little reason to believe anyone acts solely in their behalf. They respond to a sense of powerlessness by attempting to bully those they regard as having power, including health care professionals. In my experience, paradoxically, these individuals run from physicians who seek to engage with boundary clarity, despite having badgered others with constant phone calls, e-mails, and complaints. So accustomed are they to physicians holding them at arm's length and taking offense at their behavior, that they don't know what to make of one who is calling to see how they are doing and why they've missed appointments, while also not acquiescing to their demands or getting upset about them. They may wonder, "Is this person up to something . . . or could they possibly be for real?" Sometimes they will return, when they are capable of accepting help.

As a medical educator I encourage engaging with patients, starting by pointing out to students and residents when they are talking over patients' heads. When a resident asked her patient if he was having "any abdominal pain," he shook his head to indicate that he was not. I then asked the patient if he knew what "abdominal pain" is, and sheepishly he acknowledged that he did not. The resident then reframed the question avoiding medical jargon. That's just a start. When the doctor needs to be shown that the patient isn't following them, they are not engaging!

Engagement often begins with a feeling of curiosity about another person. When I meet people in social situations I'm often curious about how they think and what's important to them, but I've learned from experience to keep it light. With patients, I have the luxury of inquiring without seeming intrusive, because the information is relevant to their care. I'm often struck, however, by how often residents don't ask obvious questions. Recently a second-year resident came out of the exam room to tell me about an elderly man in a wheelchair who lives alone, has had a couple of falls, and is not controlling his diabetes. He knew how much insulin the man was taking, and what medical tests had been done to evaluate his falls. But here are things he hadn't asked: whether the man has family or friends who drop in to see him; what sorts of activities he does during the day; how he manages shopping and cooking; what he thinks or feels about his situation; how he got to his appointment that day; and what sort of work and family he had when he was younger. This may seem like a lot of information, but I've found that if you're curious and hungry for a mental picture of someone's life, you can get it in a couple of minutes in a way that feels natural.

I am not convinced by arguments that physicians don't have time to obtain psychosocial information. If you feel pressed for time, you can tell patients up front what you hope to accomplish and how much time you have. While studies of doctor-patient communication show that physicians interrupt patients too soon, I don't think that means we shouldn't interrupt at all. Patients rely on our expertise to guide the discussion, and we, not they, know how much time we have. If I'm trying to figure out if an 85-year-old man in a wheelchair who lives alone is managing okay, I'll ask him to describe how he goes shopping, prepares food, bathes, and so on. Once I've heard enough in each of these areas to know whether I should do something or not, I'll interject if needed, asking him if we can change to a different topic. Being open about the direction and goals of the conversation provides an opportunity to collaborate. If he's not able to interact this way, that's useful to know too: Is he distracted? Could he be depressed or anxious? Does he have cognitive deficits? Everything is grist for the mill. As a result, there is little unproductive time during the encounter.

This chapter is titled "Healing Interactions," rather than "Healing

Relationships" or "Healing Encounters," because it is about a way of relating in the moment even if you've never seen the person before and have little time together. My research team and I have listened to hundreds of 15- to 30-minute recorded encounters between doctors and patients, and rarely do we think to ourselves "if only they'd had more time together, they would have connected." Generally, it is the physician's behavior that determines whether the interaction sounds like a partnership to figure out what the patient needs, or a doctor trying to get through a checklist of questions and things to do. Many physicians seem to have the impression that only the latter approach is practical in the current health care climate, which judges doctors based on adherence to various care and screening guidelines, documentation requirements, and productivity. Engaging with patients, however, is not an add-on to an already long list of tasks; rather it is a nonlinear way of relating that widens the bandwidth so that more is learned and shared in the same amount of time because less is concealed.

Engaged interactions are also more personal, which is good for the doctor too. Rather than feeling drained, you feel rejuvenated because—just as you are now acknowledging another person's humanity with your attention—that person, in reciprocating, is acknowledging yours. That mutual recognition is the foundation of all healing interaction.

Questions for Reflection and Discussion

1. Can you think of a time when you felt alienated or alone, like Dr. Remen, and someone interacted with you in a way that was a breath of fresh air—that lifted your spirits and enabled you to feel more connected? If so, what was it about their behavior that had that effect? Can you give an example?

2. Do you see yourself as someone friends turn to when they are in distress or need guidance? If so, what is it that you are able to offer them that enables you to be such a valuable resource? Is that part of you accessible to your patients during medical encounters? Can you think of an example? If not, why not?

3. Have you cared for a patient like Arthur who is regarded as

difficult and manipulative? If so, what feelings did that person elicit in you? How did you process those feelings? Based on that processing, how did you respond to the individual? Did the relationship become more or less engaged and trusting? If it did not improve, do you think there is anything you could have done differently?

4. What do you do when you don't have enough time to ask a question that you think is relevant to figuring out what care and services your patient needs? How do you prioritize getting through what you want to cover versus figuring out what's really going on with them that has implications for their health? Are you able to communicate openly with them about the time constraints of the encounter so that they are best served?

5. How often do interactions with patients leave you feeling good rather than just neutral or tired? What are the characteristics of those interactions?

THREE

Your Personal Journey

You practice medicine the way you live your life.

JOHN POWELL (FORMER STUDENT OF AND LATER PHYSICIAN TO DR. AUSTER)

A T OVER 100 American medical schools, students now start their first year with a ritual called the White Coat Ceremony, which symbolizes the transition from a "lay person" to a health care professional, in a manner perhaps similar to ordination into the clergy (although that occurs at the end of schooling), or induction into the military. It's an occasion for a number of speeches, typically beginning with the dean, and then senior leaders, an inspirational speaker, and the recital of a modernized version of the Hippocratic Oath. It's also a time to generally welcome students, praise them for their accomplishments, and congratulate their parents for their children's achievements.

The inspirational speakers generally talk about the importance of listening to your patients, being compassionate and empathic, and remaining true to your ideals. What I've not heard them convey, however, is that becoming a caring, engaged healer is for most a challenging developmental process often undermined by what is called the "hidden curriculum"—the unintended lessons about what's *really* expected, typically learned from interacting with those whom students seek to emulate. What's also generally not said is that most students arrive in medical school unprepared for the relational aspects of the doctor-patient relationship and that they may never develop such capabilities. Listening to inspirational speakers, one is left with the misleading impression that the qualities they call for are guaranteed because medical students are so carefully selected. They may say, reassuringly, "You were only one of the few percent we accepted. The very fact that you are here means we have confidence that you will become a caring, compassionate physician."

A more accurate, candid White Coat Ceremony welcome, while less conventionally inspirational, might go something like this:

The things we can say for sure are that you are intelligent, have participated in a variety of extracurricular activities, are able to study hard and long, and are quite polished, particularly when interviewed. What we don't know are what demons you carry inside—in what manner you are confused or prejudiced or judgmental. We don't know which among you have an open heart and an open mind, and which have just learned to appear that way. We've done our best to screen out the latter, but medical school admissions is an imperfect process.

We also have to be candid about our own imperfections. You probably won't always be treated respectfully, and we apologize in advance for that. Sexual harassment, discriminatory behavior, and general nastiness appear to be rampant in medical education, just as they are in corporate America and in large sectors of society as a whole. This is not a sanctuary. This is the real world.

Unfortunately, you'll also see us interact with patients in ways that reflect how American medicine is generally practiced, but fall short of engaged healing interaction. We'd like to do better. While you will learn much from us, there is also much that we can learn from you. Take from us what you can in the way of knowledge and wisdom, but keep a critical eye on the unintended messages we are sending. Above all, evaluate your own behavior and reactions to patients thoughtfully.

During the early years of your training you may be in survival mode, just trying to keep it together emotionally, so that you can get through all the stuff we foist on you to memorize. We don't know if it's the right material to prepare you to be a competent doctor, although we like to believe that it is. We admit that you'll forget and won't need much of it when you practice medicine, but a fair amount of the content will be on board exams. No matter, when you get to your third year and start doing full-time clinical training, you'll begin to acquire the practical skills you need to function as a physician. You may wonder why we had you learn the sixteen different types of collagen, and we're not sure exactly; that's just the way it is. Not everything we do makes sense.

If you can forgive our limitations and accept your own, you'll be off to a good start. Some of you will sail more smoothly than others. There are students who party quite a bit and do well, and others who toil and barely get by. If you're in the former category, don't get too cocky, as the qualities required to excel as a healer rather than as just a technician have not been assessed. If you're in the latter category don't despair, for the same reasons. In the long run, the capabilities that separate students who excel on multiple-choice tests from the ones who struggle are not likely germane to caring for real patients, individuals with complex lives and personalities and often coping with chronic conditions.

What's special about the journey you are embarking on is the opportunity to grow into a person whose most valuable asset is truly wanting to figure out what's best for your patients. Such caring is expressed and relies on engaged interaction, something our culture does not encourage. And your training seems almost to discourage it. The focus is on knowing facts and completing tasks efficiently, without much attention to whether they are appropriate to the situation, or context. Much of what you are taught about the doctor-patient relationship in the classroom will also be task-based, such as how to "build rapport," and even that isn't reinforced once you start your clinical training. Unfortunately, the end result is often a disservice to patients and unhealthy for you personally.

So, how do you avoid going down such a well-trodden path in which the patient is related to, in theologian Martin Buber's terms, as "It" rather than "Thou"? Foremost, it is by remembering that you are more like your patients than otherwise. You are just a motor vehicle accident or an unlucky cancer diagnosis away from becoming a patient yourself. It will happen to you at some point if it hasn't already, hopefully later rather than sooner. Remember not to forget that, especially at today's White Coat Ceremony, so as not to think that your good fortune puts you on a higher plane than your patients. Keep in mind that the white coat is nothing other than practical outerwear. It's not a ritual object. It does have handy pockets for storing things like your stethoscope and reflex hammer. In theory, it protects your clothes and may protect patients from your clothes, but in fact hardly anyone washes it often enough to accomplish the latter. Whatever the reasons for wearing the white coat, it must never set you apart from your patients other than in the most practical sense.

It is also easy to feel as if you become a different person when you put it on—that it separates the professional you from the personal you. Open and accessible in the private sphere, you may become scripted with patients when costumed in that coat. Compartmentalizing your life that way is not good for you or your patients. So, while others will regard you as changed now that you've entered the medical profession, stay connected to yourself. And if you're not sure who you are, try to access the part of you that cares for others. If you feel like crying when you give patients bad news, you are definitely on the right track. You are becoming a healer. Good luck on your journey, which lasts a lifetime.

As a new medical school student I think I would have found such remarks helpful and more inspirational than the ones I heard. Just the fact that they could come from the leadership of a medical school would send a message that I was entering a place where it is safe and encouraged to resist conformity, question the status quo, and engage with faculty as well as fellow students. The reality, however, is that medical schools and residency programs are often a minefield for those who think differently, have difficulty meeting the narrowly constructed academic challenges, or who question standards and norms. Such a culture is likely a factor in the disproportionately high rates of burnout, depression, and suicide among students, residents, and attending physicians.

Of course there is variation in the diversity of thought and culture across medical schools and health system training environments. Some are surely healthier places to learn and work than others. But we have a long way to go. This book is about how to grow and thrive in the real world—in medicine as it is, not as we wish it were. Based on what I've experienced and observed, and through many conversations with Simon, three principles for surviving and thriving stand out. They also enable you, in the long run, to be part of the solution rather than part of the problem. The following sections introduce each of them.

"Take a Lot of Crap," but Don't Pass It On

When I was an intern, I noticed three types of responses to the 100 (and more)-hour work weeks that we endured. Surprisingly, perhaps, the most common was that nothing was wrong. These interns simply shrugged when the topic of our crazy situation came up. At the other end were those who were bitter all the time and tended to get into arguments when nurses paged at night with various requests of seemingly little urgency just when there was a chance for a bit of rest. The nurses would then complain through their managers to the intern's attending or program director who, in turn, slapped these young, angry, exhausted doctors on the wrist. The message was that we were expected not to make trouble and to suck it up.

I settled into a middle group: those who accepted our lot but didn't try to convince ourselves that what was happening was fine. A maxim that Simon taught me has served me well: *I will take a lot of crap to get what I want, but that doesn't say what I think of those who shove it in my face.* There is a lot to unpack in this expression of acceptance combined with defiance. First, that you have to know what you want to complete a difficult journey. In my case, I wanted to become a well-trained physician. Second is that in order to get to where you want to go, you have to survive the journey. Don't let anyone, including yourself, divert your mission. I think I had an advantage at internalizing this message because as a learning-disabled student I was used to assignments that made no sense and to criticism that was unhelpful. These included exams arbitrarily limited to one hour when I needed twice that time to read and digest the information, or, as a child, being told that I was unmotivated, irresponsible, and unreliable when in fact I was desperate to learn but simply overwhelmed. Initially I responded by acting out. I recall an incident in math class in seventh grade when the teacher grilled me in front of my classmates, triggering confusion and panic to the point where I had to admit I couldn't say whether 70 or 80 came first. Hoping for some positive attention, I intentionally fell out of my chair. Instead, I was kicked out of class. Over the subsequent years, however, as my desire to become a physician became a single-minded focus, I learned how to adapt to situations where my learning disability put me or others at risk. For instance, during internship I realized that after 35 hours without sleep I couldn't catch prescription errors, so I showed all my scripts to a colleague before signing them. Frankly, I wondered if anyone should be writing prescriptions on no sleep, but knew I was not in a position to challenge the status quo. In short, I learned that the first order of business is survival, not rebellion.

Perhaps worse than screwing up prescriptions because of fatigue is attempting procedures unsupervised before you are ready, out of a fear of looking look bad if you ask for help. "See one, do one, teach one" is a dangerous old saying among house staff. For instance, we learned to put large catheters into patients' necks, often late at night with on-the-job training from residents who had recently been trained themselves. We each carried around logbooks that indicated the number of times one had to complete a procedure supervised before one could do it independently or teach others. There was no gold standard assessment about whether any of us were doing it correctly. But there was pressure to get the job done without needing help. As a result, patients were sometimes subjected to numerous large-bore needle sticks in the neck by an inexperienced trainee who didn't want to look bad, with potentially lifelong complications. I made a decision on the first day of internship that I would never cover up my inexperience at a cost to a patient. Hence I asked questions or called for assistance often. It did come with a price. I recall a supervising resident saying to me, "Saul, you know you are not where you should be at this stage in your training." Hearing that didn't feel good, but the alternative would have felt worse. I will "take a lot of crap . . ."

And finally, third, complying with expectations does not mean buying into the system or idealizing the people who perpetuate it. Beware the "Stockholm syndrome," in which the kidnapped adopt the ideology of their captors, lest you become part of the dysfunctional status quo yourself. A few years after I finished my residency there was a national movement to regulate training work hours. It didn't come from within the profession, which lacked the good sense to reform itself, but from the federal government. In fact, quite a few medical education leaders resisted change. Even some residents complained that reducing the hours they worked per week would compromise their education. This despite an avalanche of evidence that sleep deprivation diminishes learning and performance. The organization that accredits residency programs finally took reform seriously after Congress threatened to intervene if it didn't. I was a residency director at that point. To me the need for reform was clear, but to many others it was not. Having bought into a pernicious culture, they were apologists for it. That attitude is neither good for patients nor the trainees who follow in their teachers' footsteps.

Strive to Succeed, but Don't Fear Failure

My first year of medical school was academically the most challenging for me. I worked all the time—not to excel, just to pass. Nevertheless, I failed my first anatomy exam. On Friday or Saturday evenings, when other students were partying or relaxing in front of the TV, I was studying. I thought my chances of making it through the first year were reasonable, but not certain.

An epiphany I had one evening was that if I flunked out, I'd still be okay, even though it would mean not becoming a doctor and having to find something else to do. In other words, I discovered that my basic sense of well-being was not reliant on achieving a career aspiration. Although I was consumed *with* becoming a physician, I had not been consumed *by* it. This perspective was grounding. One might think it's foolhardy to contemplate failure when one is striving to succeed. However, learning to separate who I am from what I am trying to do enabled me to focus on the latter. Becoming a doctor was simply something that I as a person wanted to accomplish. Now it was just a matter of saying *"I will take a lot of crap to get what I want . . ."*

I shared this insight about being okay with failure in a short essay I published in 2002, in the journal *Academic Medicine*, titled "Learning Medicine with a Learning Disability: Reflections of a Survivor." The piece was based on a talk I gave to a class of first-year medical students at Simon's invitation. Simon was teaching a class titled "Human Context in Health Care" at the nation's only military medical school, the Uniformed Services University of the Health Sciences. Regular panel discussions, often featuring physicians talking about challenges that were intensely personal, reflected the trust we all had in Simon creating a safe space. I was on a panel with two other physicians with disabilities: one was quadriplegic from a rugby accident that occurred while he was in medical school, and the other had a renal transplant as a result of a rare kidney disease. We were looking up at a couple hundred first-year students in military uniform, in a steeply angled auditorium. Sitting between these two guys I remember thinking to myself, "Wow, do I have it that bad?" Interestingly, after I spoke I got the sense they were looking at me sympathetically and asking themselves the same question!

While I was preparing for that presentation, Simon coached me to be unsparingly honest about my disability. I found that tough to do now that I'd "made it." Having completed my training and passed my board certification exams, there was a desire to hide from others that part of who I am. The reality, however, is that I was as learning disabled then— and still am now—as during the years when I had to struggle to keep afloat academically as a student myself, and that can be hard to admit. I still have a recurring dream that I'm back in college and medical school, as a middle-aged adult with the training I have now, taking all those classes all over again. My classmates don't know that I have twenty-five years of practice experience under my belt. I do well, without much effort, and enjoy the experience. But, when I wake up, I wonder what it would really be like if I went back to the first year of medical school, and I think that it would probably be as difficult now as it was then.

In my essay about my learning disability I wrote, "I came to accept that I would be okay even if I did fail. I confronted the possibility of failure and considered the worst possible case scenario, which was that

I would not get to be a physician. I realized that as much as I did not want that to happen and would do everything in my power to keep it from happening, I would still be okay if I failed. Accepting myself in that way was essential in an environment that challenged who I was and still am."

More than 15 years later I still get notes of appreciation from premedical students, medical students, and residents who have come across my essay during a difficult time. They tell me how affirming it's been to read about what seemed like their own personal travail. Often they are in a precarious situation, struggling to remain in school or a residency program, feeling misunderstood and judged by their teachers and supervisors. The most recent letter I received was from an internal medicine resident who described how her marginalization as a learning disabled physician who'd failed one of the licensure exams because she couldn't get through all the questions in time, was exacerbated by her status as an international medical graduate. She mentioned my comment about recognizing that I'd be okay even if I failed as an important source of strength for her. She too was determined not to conflate multiple-choice test performance with self-worth.

Answering the question "If I can't be a doctor, then who am I?" is just as important if you do succeed. Some years ago I mentored a struggling medical student who would just shudder when I posed it to him. The possibility was unthinkable. He was the son of immigrants, raised by a single mother in poverty, with self-imposed expectations that he make his family proud. We got acquainted when I mentioned my learning disability to a group of students I was teaching. He came up to me afterward and said, "I think I have what you have." Jason and I kept in close touch for 10 years as he struggled to clear huge hurdles: repeating a couple of years of medical school, retaking medical licensure exams, and then retaking board exams several times. As all too often happens, the certifying bodies that administer the tests would not acknowledge his disability despite ample documentation, so he was unable to get the extra time on exams that would constitute appropriate accommodations. He pushed himself unrelentingly, however, eventually completing medical school and residency and then going on to obtain additional training and certification in one of the elite subspecialties at a famous hospital. He was obsessively conscientious at one of the busiest and best centers in the nation. I often thought that if I or a member of my family needed the expertise Jason had acquired, he'd be the one I'd trust, given how meticulous and skillful he had become. He illustrated the disconnect between what's measured and what matters in health care.

Despite "making it," however, Jason was neither content nor collegial in the work environment, likely out of intense insecurity. There were allegations of harassment, bullying, and arrogance. Privately he expressed remorse and worked hard to "lay low" so as to avoid conflict. But he struggled to find a way to engage positively with colleagues despite the warmth and openness I saw him show in the private sphere. He had to force himself to act "nice" at work where he felt scrutinized, to restrain his tendency to say things that could get him into trouble. I had the frustrating sense that while Jason persevered in the face of daunting obstacles, he was not able to grow from the experience personally. Jason couldn't respect himself without external validation. I cringed when he shared with me that he had told his mother on her deathbed that he'd passed his boards when he hadn't yet. His sense of self-worth was reliant on being—or at least appearing—successful. Eventual success did not bring him peace of mind. He seemed increasingly paranoid, cynical, and embittered. His personal journey to becoming a physician had hollowed him.

What are the lessons here for those medical students and residents, perhaps a majority, who rarely if ever fear flunking out? You are fortunate, but, given the prevailing culture, the risk of defining yourselves by your grades, board exams, performance evaluations, and the validation of peers and superiors remains. In the process it's easy to forget what it's all about. A sense of connection with patients, joy in one's work, and the actual quality of one's care are hardly in the mix. By the time training is complete, too much operant conditioning has taken place. Medical training is all-consuming, and as the investment in effort and time grows, so do the potential gains and losses. You become expert at hanging in there, year after year and stage after stage, even if it feels empty inside. At each point you master what's expected to do well. There is a hierarchy and a power structure, and you know your place. The incentives are always to conform, which means that you work in an environment where the range of normative behaviors is quite narrow. You are judged by what your peers and professors think of you, not what your patients are experiencing.

Conformity can be an asset to patient care in that it reinforces some desirable traits, like showing up on time, dressing appropriately, acquiring expected knowledge, exhibiting accepted social norms. But it also has drawbacks. First, conforming makes you narrow-minded. For instance, you'll look up the latest guidelines for managing hyperlipidemia because your supervisors value that information. However, figuring out why a patient keeps coming back with vague complaints as if they are looking for something but can't tell you what may not count for much. As a result, you may be less interested in finding answers, even though doing so would be better for your patients and probably more rewarding.

Second, conforming too much fosters insecurity, as your capacity to listen to and trust yourself remains underdeveloped. You become thin-skinned when people with less power challenge you. For instance, you may not like it when patients look things up on the Internet, thinking "Who's the one who went to medical school here?" And yet there are numerous examples of patients contributing to their own care by finding vital information their doctor overlooked.

The antidote is realizing that your values are even more important than your success, as others define it. The affirmation that "I will be okay even if I fail," at the earliest stages of one's training, amounts to another way of saying, "I'm not defined by how others measure me," leaving room for independence of thought, a willingness to question norms, and the courage to engage, diminishing the chance that you'll evolve into a burned-out task completer.

Stay Focused, but Don't Lose Your Curiosity

Taking a lot of crap without becoming embittered and learning to live with fear of failure give you resilience and self-confidence. They are an essential foundation, but they don't propel you forward developmentally. That requires curiosity.

I think of myself as a curious person, but I suppressed this quality during medical school and residency training so that I could focus on absorbing the information that was required, which for me was all-consuming. This didn't come naturally, as I've often been more interested in things that I don't have to know than the things that are expected for school or work. When I was in seventh grade and struggling academically, one of my history teachers wrote home to my parents that "Saul seems to prefer the recommended to the required reading." That was probably because the required reading was often didactic, packed with dates and events, such as what you'd find in a textbook, whereas the optional material was more narrative or exploratory, such as a historical novel or a primary-source document. I'm sure I wasn't the only one more drawn to the latter. Nevertheless, my curiosity posed a threat to my academic success.

In medical school, academic survival sometimes required choosing rote memorization over understanding. I remember in renal physiology finding the kidney to be both fascinating and perplexing. Our professor was the author of the textbook we used, which seemed quite lucid. However, as soon as I started to look at the test questions from prior years' exams, I realized that I would never be able to answer them based on fundamental principles. They were too esoteric. So I memorized responses based on old tests, and passed the exams. When I was reminiscing about this time in my life with a colleague, she said she remembered an exam in which the anatomy professor put a clavicle on the table apart from the rest of the cadaver, and asked students to ascertain whether it was the right or left clavicle, what each side would be connected to, and the correct orientation were it actually positioned in the body. When would a physician need to know what to do with a fully detached clavicle? Given that there are around 206 bones and 650 muscles, not to mention organs, tendons, and large nerves—and that anatomy is just one of several courses taken during a semester—the faculty could really mess with our minds. And yet we prevailed, at least on paper: I remember studying one night using flash cards I'd made for a neurophysiology test and realizing I had no idea what the terms on either side of the cards meant, but was confident that if asked about what was on one side, I should respond with whatever was on the other. I did fine on the test—but felt frustrated because I had a real desire to learn.

During internship there wasn't much time for curiosity either. A post-call day ended when all patients were "tucked in," meaning we'd addressed all acute issues that had brought them into the hospital the prior night. Post-call house staff also had to complete all the discharge paperwork for patients who were going home. A key variable that determined how long we'd be there was the number of patients who were assigned to us, which was determined by whom we had admitted on call. Since we were on call every third or fourth night, it was imperative to get patients out quickly, or one's service would grow to an unmanageable size.

Post-call days were a race to get patients out the door as fatigue threatened to overwhelm me after 36–40 hours on my feet. Often I'd have to do a couple of procedures, such as a paracentesis—drawing fluid out of a patient's abdomen—or putting a central line in someone's groin or neck. There might also be a family meeting that included social workers, home care staff, and the patient's closest kin. Throughout, my pager would go off every of couple of minutes with requests from nurses and technicians to put in orders or to come and evaluate a problem. From time to time, a patient admitted the previous night was too medically unstable to keep on my service, and I'd have to transfer them to an intensive care unit, where another team would take over. Although it meant they were seriously ill, I felt relief because of the reduced stress and workload—as perverse as that may seem.

Given the pace, I avoided doing anything I didn't have to. There were many opportunities to indulge my curiosity that I decided to forgo. In particular, I wondered how various tests that I ordered for my patients were done, such as those in the cardiology laboratory or in interventional radiology. When my patients needed a surgical procedure, I thought about following them into the operating room to observe. Such firsthand knowledge might make me a better doctor, deepening my understanding of the risks and benefits, including the discomfort and pain patients experienced from the various orders I placed. I have the impression that some of my fellow residents did occasionally observe specialists caring for their patients. Nevertheless, I rarely broke from the routine of getting mine in and out the door, handling crises when they occurred, and writing all my notes as fast as possible so that I could get some sleep before returning early the next morning to begin another cycle.

While following my patients into the lab or operating room was not enticing enough to lengthen my day, I did make time for patients and families when complex dynamics arose, such as dissatisfaction with their care, anger and discord derailing decision making, or confusion and grief about what was happening when a patient was acutely ill. I was drawn to the challenge and creativity required to respond to these situations, as much as I dreaded them. Walking into a room that is tense with angry family members who don't know you but have had several frustrating encounters with other doctors and staff requires intense concentration. One has to calibrate what one says to the tenor of the group, and through careful questioning figure out the text and the subtext of what is going on. Being completely present and open with people who are suspicious and in distress about the care of their loved one is essential. Almost invariably these situations had reached a boiling point because of the missteps of others who had reacted defensively or dismissively to a family's complaints.

I have become adept at engaging with distressed patients and families, in part because I have found a way to be myself rather than retreat into a defensive mode or adopt a persona. I've learned that how a clinician responds to these situations can have a profound effect on their outcome. Good outcomes, such as resolution of a breakdown in trust between a family and the health care team, are truly satisfying. I've thought a lot about how to walk into interpersonal conflict, remaining attentive to each individual's boundaries while openly engaged. It's a challenge that's interested me.

While curiosity is invaluable to growing as a physician, it is fragile. If it gets in the way of succeeding at something important to us, we can suppress it. On the other hand, if it pulls us in a direction that is affirming or gives us pleasure, we will find ways to indulge it. Curiosity is so important not only because it leads us to discover new things and solve problems we otherwise would have overlooked, but because it is so close to caring. "To be curious" is almost synonymous with "to care." Both feel like an inner impulse that draws us forward out of desire. When you don't care or are not curious, you'll still do things out of a sense of responsibility, fear of reprisal, or mere routine, but only with a sense of being dragged forward or along, rather than setting the course. Curiosity and caring stave off indifference and burnout.

Where Are You on Your Journey?

So, then, these are the questions you may ask yourself: Are you able to put up with a lot of crap to get what you want without buying into the status quo? While trying your best to succeed in your career, can you appreciate that who you are does not depend on it? Does curiosity help sustain you in your daily work, especially in interactions with patients?

For the first, unfortunately, I've seen colleagues behave disrespectfully toward medical students, residents, and junior faculty despite— or perhaps because of—how they were treated during their training years. A fourth-year medical student I got to know was required to prove that his grandfather had died to postpone taking an end of clerkship exam so he could travel out of town to the funeral. He felt humiliated. What was the point? Had the physician teaching the class been treated that way once? What does it take to break cycles of abuse? First, it takes calling it what it is and rejecting perpetuation. Second, it is discovering that treating underlings respectfully is far more enjoyable and productive. I've found it richly rewarding to see students, young physicians, and others thrive when they work in an appreciative, supportive environment. I trust them unless they give me a reason not to. And, third, it's less stressful to treat everyone as an equal because that is, in fact, what they are. Medicine is hierarchical, and some of that is for good reason. As the attending physician, I am legally and ethically responsible for the patients that medical students and residents who report to me care for. Hence, I make the final decisions, and they must respect that. But as *people*, we are equals. They should feel comfortable telling me when they think I'm wrong. By doing so they are contributing to our shared mission of helping patients get the best care. If I make them uncomfortable, then I am not serving our patients.

For me, creating a positive work environment has no downside. However, I didn't always think that way. As noted earlier, I used to react with indignation when I thought my subordinates were not according me some deference, as when a resident addressed me as "Hey, Saul." Fortunately, Simon pointed out that this was a sign that they were comfortable with me, not disrespectful. I needed someone else to clarify boundaries, as I was unable to distinguish what was going on in my insecure head from what was actually taking place. I cannot count the number of times I've benefited from this lesson. For instance, years later, I moved into an administrative position in which a staff person who reported to me suffered chronic intermittent depression and was frequently irritable. She was also highly competent when at her best. As she became increasingly comfortable that I was safe, she started to berate me about all sorts of things. On the one hand it felt unfair because I was her strongest advocate, which should have been obvious to her. On the other hand I appreciated that she needed to vent and trusted that I would not act vindictively. She showed her appreciation in unexpected ways. One day she picked up a large manuscript I was working on, took it home over the weekend, and meticulously edited it. The job was completely outside of her assigned duties. I think it was partly her way of reciprocating and partly what made her an asset in the first place: if she thought she could help out with something she took the initiative.

The benefits of fostering a supportive work environment go beyond the practical to the existential. None of us is around that long, and nearly all are forgotten. What impact do we have? When people feel respected and supportive they, in turn, treat others well. It has a ripple effect that pushes back on all the negativity in the world. This is not an abstraction. If you are able to break a dysfunctional cycle one relationship at a time, there is an immeasurable multiplier effect. Your legacy is transformative.

For the second question above—the one about not living constrained by fear of failure—I've had the advantage of failing often enough as a result of my learning disability to know I'll be okay. Most people who get into medical school have a long track record of academic excellence. Success came relatively easily to them starting at an early age. Not so for those of us with learning disabilities. For years I'd noticed how hard I worked compared to my classmates who did better anyway. I asked myself, "Am I just not bright?" At the same time I acknowledged there was more to me than my struggles in school. By the time I got to medical school I'd come to appreciate that I was an odd mix of intellect, talent, and ineptitude. The curriculum and culture seemed specially designed to bring out the latter. The poor fit between what I had to offer and what the educational program valued in the first two years gave me an outsider's perspective. If I had been a great student, it would have been easy to embrace everything about medical training, sort of the way those with inherited wealth who just keep getting richer tend to favor the status quo in America despite rampant inequality.

Admittedly my critique of medical education could also be self-serving, as a rationale for not being a great student. Even if there is something to that argument, I think that learning not to rely on external validation is essential to growth as a healer. That is because much of what matters is rarely measured or observed. As researchers, I and my team have carried out studies in which actors portraying "mystery patients" see multiple doctors while following the same script. The physicians agree, in advance, not to know when they are interacting with a fake patient who is recording the visit. We've documented enormous variation in the quality of care different doctors provide. Most of it is currently not measured by auditors that monitor the medical record, because collecting the data requires covertly observing the encounter. For instance, one doctor might be conscientious when helping a patient who is unsure about how to take a medication correctly, but sloppy when it comes to documenting all the care they provided. Another doctor might do the reverse—meticulous with the medical record but sloppy with the patient. We've noticed that many who are like the latter exaggerate what they do, checking off boxes for services they barely—if at all—provided, like performing a review of systems. Who do you think is going to go on record as the better physician? Which one is better for patients and US health care? And, finally, if you had to choose, which one would you rather be?

I don't mean to imply that overcoming fear of failure is the only path to becoming an independent thinker who does the right thing when no one is watching. Simon was a superb student, at the top of his class during his medical school years. Yet, as a doctor he instinctively put patient care ahead of looking good. For instance, he was always behind on writing his notes and even got reprimanded for not getting them done on schedule. Not to excuse such delinquency, but I'm sure he spent more time than most actually helping patients. A remarkable, albeit extreme, example comes to mind: One afternoon he was meeting with a patient who also happened to be a senior administrator at the medical center, and it came out that he was suicidal. When asked, the man acknowledged that he owned several guns. Simon stood up and said, "Let's go get them." He drove the man to his house, picked up the weapons, and put them in the trunk of his car. Weeks later, when his patient was no longer at risk, Simon returned them.

I'm not endorsing Simon's approach, as he put himself in legal jeopardy by driving around with weapons he didn't own and was not licensed to carry. In addition to his medical training he also has a law degree, so he was not unaware of the consequences. They just weren't as important to him as keeping his patient safe and protecting his reputation in an environment where secrets travel fast. Other physicians might have taken a more conventional tack, such as attempting to include family, law enforcement, or another physician who could commit the patient to inpatient care to prevent a tragedy. But Simon's patient had a relatively high profile in a tight-knit military community, and he wanted to spare the man any humiliation or harm to his reputation. His intervention accomplished all that. It's not likely a plan that would have crossed Simon's mind, however, if he thought conventionally and was afraid of taking risks.

While I don't recommend breaking the law to care for your patients, I do recommend keeping stories like this one in mind as models for how to think about patient care. Simon once said, "I would stand on my head if it would help my patients." It took me a while to understand what he was getting at. His point is that we shouldn't constrain ourselves to what's in our medical tool kit. We're there to help our patients with their health and health care. To do that effectively we need to be thinking about how we—based on whatever distinct qualities we have—can be helpful to them, rather than just relying on what we're trained to do in our formal medical education.

A small number of physicians do quietly work this way. While my team has never recorded a physician actually standing on their head during a visit—and I can't think of a reason why that would benefit anyone—one of our mystery patients who portrayed a man with chronic back pain was touched when a doctor got down on the floor and demonstrated each of the exercises he should do, unaware that he was not a real patient. It was an unselfconscious, pragmatic, caring response that would have gone undetected in a professional assessment of the physician's skills. His behavior stood out from that of the other physicians who saw the same patient and simply handed him preprinted instructions on how to do back exercises. The physician was focused on helping, even if it meant stepping outside of the expected conventions of a doctor-patient encounter. Most physicians we hear stick to what is safe and predictable, rather than try something new to help a patient. This physician, however, evidently wasn't inhibited by fears of looking silly or unprofessional by getting down on the exam room floor. I believe that's what Simon meant by saying he would "stand on his head."

Finally, for the third principle, the question is whether you are curious about the people you care for. And if you've lost your curiosity, is it extinguished or suppressed? Curiosity has been described as the motivation to reduce uncertainty. If you're not sure why your patient isn't following the care plan as directed, for instance, you could ask them. If you are not curious, you may simply lecture them about why they need to do better. This approach, however, requires making assumptions that can be mistaken. For instance, when I was teaching a group of fourth-year medical students, we met a woman on the inpatient unit who had been admitted four times for missing hemodialysis. Nobody had asked her why. Each time she was told how dangerous her behavior was and not to miss dialysis again. It turned out she was missing dialysis to take a grandson with chronic illness to his doctor visits. Her dialysis site was far from the pediatrics clinic where her grandson received his care. She could schedule a Medicaid van to transport her to either location from her home, but not to both. She prioritized his health over hers. Once we knew what was going on, we arranged for her dialysis to occur at the same hospital as his clinic appointments so she didn't have to choose between them. She never missed dialysis again.

Why hadn't anybody wondered what led a seemingly reasonable woman to act in an apparently irrational manner at risk to herself? Rather than exhibiting such curiosity, it appears her physicians just assumed she had an attitude problem. Each admission note documented that they'd advised her of the consequences of missing hemodialysis, but not that they'd looked for a cause.

A curious doctor would have asked the evident question: "Ms. Garcia, why do you keep missing your dialysis?" The fact that so many made the same assumption about her leads to the following question: Would they more likely have wondered what was going on had Ms. Garcia been an educated, upper-middle-class, Caucasian woman coming repeatedly to the emergency department after missing her hemodialysis? Beware of bias suppressing curiosity.

What can one do to avoid making false assumptions about people? Most directly, by challenging one's own preconceptions. Regarding Ms. Garcia it would be to ask oneself, "What are the possible circumstances of this woman's life that might account for her missing dialysis?" Starting from the perspective that we all have reasons for doing what we do, albeit sometimes misguided, enables physicians to think and explore rather than to presume and assume that they know why a patient has made a specific choice or set of choices that don't seem to make sense.

Without curiosity about their patients, physicians may be providing technically competent care, but often without giving their patients what they need. It is a self-inflicted, monotonous, and emotionally depleting way to practice because of the absence of a human connection. Relating to patients in such a detached manner starts early. Simon recalled an incident that occurred when he was teaching a second-year student to take a medical history: The prior evening the course director had identified a 62-year-old man who said he'd be happy to participate in a practice interview. However, when Simon and the student arrived that morning, the man seemed distracted. As the student began to question him he responded tersely and with little interest. The student nevertheless forged ahead, trying to make his way through each component of a medical history. As he struggled, the atmosphere in the room became increasingly oppressive. Simon finally considered it imperative to intervene. Interrupting, he said, "You seem upset. Is there something bothering you?" The patient explained that he was told the evening before that he would be discharged that afternoon, and had arranged for a friend to take him home, but shortly before Simon and the student arrived, he learned he would have to stay another day. He felt some urgency about notifying his friend, who would have to leave work early to get to the hospital on time, and he hadn't yet been able to reach him. However, he did not want to break his commitment to meet with the student. Simon replied that reaching his friend was the more urgent need, and that other arrangements could be made for the student. The patient's tense demeanor at once dissolved. He shook their hands as they left, and took out his phone.

As soon as they'd left the room, the student looked amazedly at Simon and exclaimed, "Wow! How did you do that? I tried so hard to connect with him and you knew what to say immediately." Simon replied, "If he had been your friend looking that upset, wouldn't you have asked him the same question?" As if a light bulb had suddenly gone on, the student asked, "You mean you talk to patients like you talk to people?" What's remarkable to me about this example is not the awkward interview—I see or hear that sort of thing all the time—it's the student's candidness about his own distorted perspective. It is a first step to opening up and beginning to engage.

These three principles are a foundation for growth and a bulwark against conformity, but just a beginning. The first (*taking a lot of crap but not passing it on*) enables us to survive in difficult work environments without becoming bitter or vindictive. The second (*striving to succeed but not fearing failure*) grounds us if we are struggling so that our core sense of well-being is not dependent on external measures of success. The third (*staying focused but not losing our curiosity*) gives us joy by keeping us engaged in our work and continuously learning and growing.

With sufficient grounding and curiosity, each of us can find the courage and honesty to acknowledge, at least to ourselves, where we are developmentally in our journey to becoming healers. This requires self-reflection. I wish I could say that the socialization process of medical training is the sole cause of the detachment and lack of curiosity and engagement that are so prevalent among physicians. Unfortunately, many who enter the profession bring these deficits with them. In particular, they have learned to fear engagement. Parents or others with power over them may have related to them in ways that discouraged being open and vulnerable. Spanking a child, for instance, is always a violation of personal boundaries, yet it still occurs. Many of us were spanked or verbally disparaged by those who had power over us. Whether we recognize it or not, these experiences have a lasting effect.

Although not knowing how to relate to people with an openness about who you are and a respect for who they are imposes a lifelong psychic burden, in the practice of medicine it is a professional liability. Acquiring the capacity to engage with boundary clarity is the essential personal journey all physicians must traverse, with a rich payoff in both their personal and professional spheres. Depending on where you are starting from, the journey may entail giving up pretensions, presumptions, posturing, and fears, so as to recognize your shared humanity in all interactions. It is the practitioner's personal qualities, rather than a set of skills, that make a healer.

Questions for Reflection and Discussion

1. How have you been affected by the stress of your medical training? Has it helped you grow into a better physician and/or might it be limiting or even undermining the qualities that you would want most in someone who is your doctor?

2. How has your medical education journey enabled you to develop as a person? In what ways might it have impeded you, if any? How has your training impacted the way you relate to friends, family, and patients? Are the changes similar or different across these three groups? In what ways?

3. What do you see as particular strengths of your personality and character that benefit your patients the most? What are some of the ways in which you think you may need to grow to become the kind of physician your patients most need?

4. If you flunked out of medical school or residency, what would you most want to do instead? How would it be similar or different from what you have sought in a medical career? Can you draw connections between your second choice and medicine to gain perspective on what you most love to do? Assuming you stay in medicine, how can you be sure you are most likely to find it?

5. What's happened to your curiosity during medical training? What are you more curious about? What are you less curious about? Specifically, what questions do you find yourself asking or wanting to ask as you go through the day? How do you think your curiosity or lack of curiosity affects how you relate to and care for your patients and how you feel about your work?

FOUR

Overcoming Judgmentalism

In our lives, we do the best we can with what we've got. Our choices may seem strange to others—funny, frightening, or simply stupid—but in the balance of our lives, as we see it, those are the choices that make the most sense.

SIMON AUSTER

D URING MY first few years as an attending physician, supervising a team of residents and medical students on the wards of an urban public hospital several months each year, I was often irritated or frustrated with patients. Almost all were poor, and most were Latinx or African American. Twenty years later I can barely remember what I was upset about, as I don't have those feelings anymore. I think I perceived many as ungrateful, malingering, or uncooperative. I hid these sentiments during patient interactions, but they did spill over in comments I made about patients with the residents on my team.

Such a negative, judgmental attitude was cultivated during my own training. For instance, as an intern I simultaneously admired and was horrified by a brilliant, charismatic senior resident who sometimes disparaged patients behind their backs. This guy was a walking *Harrison's Principles of Internal Medicine* who had authored a paper in a renowned medical journal, so lack of intelligence was not his problem. I remember hearing him describe how he got rid of a patient in the emergency department (ED) seeking to be admitted with a variety of complaints who he believed was malingering. It's possible the man had nowhere else safe to go on a winter night. This resident recounted how he walked into the enclosed bay in the ED with a nasogastric tube draped casually around his neck along with his stethoscope, and said,

"I think we're going have to use an extra-large catheter today to take a sample of urine from you." Not surprisingly, the man took one look at the large-bore tube, intended to go down an esophagus, not a narrow penile ureter, and left as soon as possible. As this story was related to us over dinner in the residents' conference room, everyone laughed.

Looking back, I'm ashamed that I was not immune to such a judgmental attitude. I have, however, since recognized the harm of making negative assumptions about patients and then reacting to them based on those unsubstantiated beliefs. There is of course the indignity, disrespect, dishonesty, and breach of fiduciary responsibility involved in misleading a patient because you judge them unworthy of your services, as in the example above. Less often recognized, however, is that judging also extinguishes thinking. Once we conclude that a teenage girl on her third pregnancy is "irresponsible," that a patient who doesn't work and misses appointments is "lazy," that a patient who continues to smoke despite emphysema is "weak," or in this case, that a man in the emergency room with puzzling complaints is malingering, we are no longer inclined to find out or even wonder what is really going on.

Once we pass judgment, we cease to exercise judgment. I recall a young couple, struggling to care for a 15-month-old son with congenital anomalies including a cleft palate, who had missed numerous doctor appointments. The toddler had been hospitalized because of failure to thrive. The state authorities (Department of Child and Family Services, DCFS) evaluated the family situation and, along with the inpatient care team, arrived at a plan with the parents that they must not miss any follow-up appointments following discharge. That was a lot to expect, since the child had scheduled visits with a craniofacial specialist, developmental pediatrics, occupational therapy, physical therapy, and general outpatient primary care, among others. Following discharge the family missed just one of them. The resident notified DCFS and then called me to say that "DCFS will probably take the child." This despite a recent note in the patient's medical record, just three days prior, documenting that the little boy was doing just fine.

What the resident didn't do before calling DCFS was contact the family and find out why they missed that appointment. There were possible explanations other than neglect, given the other stresses on the parents. In addition to their young child with complex medical needs, the parents had two other children, the father worked, English was a second language, and the family was quite poor with limited resources for transportation. Furthermore, the resident had not taken into account that a specialist had just evaluated the child and documented that he was thriving. Fortunately, we were able to intervene with DCFS, and the child stayed with his parents and continued to do well.

Physicians can be unabashed about being judgmental. A senior resident in our clinic saw a man with a heroin addiction who had been diagnosed with a lung mass based on a CT scan at another hospital. The resident asked the patient to request a copy of the films and bring them to his next appointment. He returned a couple weeks later without the films, saying that the hospital wanted $20 to print out the images, which he said was money he didn't have. The resident told the patient that he couldn't help him until he got those films. When I asked why he didn't just contact the hospital directly to fax over the reports, he replied, "If that man can't forgo the cost of a little bit of heroin to pay for those films, his life isn't worth saving." When I commented that that was judgmental, he shrugged and replied, "Everyone is judgmental." Needless to say, we contacted the hospital and got those films.

What does it mean, exactly, to judge someone? Law and religion are the two formalized systems for rendering judgment. In jurisprudence it refers to the determination of guilt or innocence as defined by the rules that govern a particular society. These are laws created by humans for the purpose of maintaining a safe and orderly place to live. A person who violates them is a criminal. In a theological context, a person who commits an offense against a religious law that is believed to come from God is a sinner. Anyone other than a judge or god who judges is simply "judgmental."

Hence, when we say someone is judgmental, we mean that this individual is judging others without any legitimate reason for doing so, often assigning labels such as "irresponsible," "careless," or "lazy." These are critiques of the person, not just their actions. A lazy man is expected to continue to avoid work. A careless individual is expected to remain unreliable. Such judgments diminish a person's value in the eyes of whoever is doing the judging, as we saw in the case of the resident who didn't feel the drug addict was worthy of help.

Being judgmental is antithetical to healing for at least three reasons. First, when you judge someone, you are making an assumption about them that may not be correct—for instance, that they don't take their medication because they are irresponsible, when in fact the underlying problem is that they can't afford to. Second, once you attribute a behavior to a character trait, you cease to ask questions because you think you already have the answers. Once you decide a patient is just "non-compliant," you're even less likely to find out what really accounts for their behavior. And third, to judge another is to assume a godlike superiority that undermines engagement—a form of interaction that can only occur when two people are on a level playing field.

There is also a fundamental illogic behind being judgmental. To judge someone is to believe that they are the primary cause of their actions, which is never the case. An emotionally unstable parent who is negligent did not choose the genes, family they were born into, violent neighborhood in which they were raised or other factors beyond their control that made them an unsuitable caretaker at a particular moment in time. One might respond, "Well, I know other people who grew up in tough, unfortunate circumstances and turned out all right." But that is missing the point. If they turned out all right, something must have been different, either at the level of their genes or chance factors during their upbringing, such as a nurturing teacher or neighbor, or some other positive influence. The notion that we can somehow rise above our genetic potential and the environment into which we are born and raised is magical thinking. It is a deeply held belief that leads us to pass judgment.

It is hard not to be judgmental unless you let the belief go. For those who need empirical evidence that we are not in control, functional MRI studies demonstrate that the outcome of a decision is encoded in the prefrontal and parietal cortices up to 10 seconds before it enters awareness, that is, before we "decide" to act. One can only speculate about why the fallacy is so deeply embedded in our belief system, but I suspect it's because we sure feel as if we're in control. From moment to moment we perceive we're making decisions about what we're going to eat, when to take our medications, or whether to rob a bank. The thought that neurons fire based on genetic instructions and all previous life experience up to the present instant is, for many, disconcerting to contemplate. However, if you're trying to understand or influence another's behavior, it is essential to appreciate that every action is a reaction to myriad factors, including a person's upbringing, current environment, past traumas and chance events that collectively make up the context for what you are observing.

Of course, you'll never be able to fully explain or predict a person's behavior no matter how well you know them, but social science and psychology research have yielded many insights about correlations. Adverse childhood events (ACEs), including physical or sexual abuse, or incarceration of a parent during childhood, are strong predictors of physical, emotional, and behavioral problems later in life. We also know that concomitant affirming relationships, such as with a caring teacher, physician, or neighbor can mitigate the adverse long-term effects of childhood traumas. To disregard all this information—to not consider a patient's life context—and to conclude instead that their poor life choices, such as getting pregnant at an early age, simply reflect "carelessness" is judgmental.

Once we recognize that there is a story behind why a teenage patient had three babies at such an early age, and that she didn't get to write that story—only to live it—we can engage. The purpose of engaging is not to understand why, as even she is unlikely to have a complete explanation, but to understand what to do about it. If the mother just needs a helping hand, you will do what you can to get her the needed services. In the clinic where I work we have special programs for teenage and low-income parents that include home visits and parenting classes. If her mental health is fraying, you'll treat her condition, if doing so is within the scope of your practice, or refer her to someone who can.

How does one remain nonjudgmental when a patient is harming others, such as when they perpetrate child abuse? In such situations, I find it helpful to think of individuals as *accountable* rather than *re-*

sponsible for their actions. An abuser may have suffered untold abuse themselves, and aggression may be the only way in which they know how to react to stress and conflict in parenting relationships. In this context they are no more responsible for their actions than a ball is responsible for breaking a window. Nevertheless they must be held to account for their actions in order to maintain a safe and orderly society. Trained and authorized individuals should make a determination about whether the parents will lose custody based on an assessment of the risks and benefits to their offspring.

The shift from thinking about the person to thinking about the consequences of their actions primes us to ask, "What harm might they cause?" and "What can I can do to mitigate that harm while remaining mindful of unintended consequences?" I've seen well-intentioned physicians shy away from such questions because they mistakenly thought that asking them was in itself judgmental. A resident I was supervising in the pediatrics clinic decided not to notify the DCFS about an emotionally unstable mother, despite ample evidence that her children were at risk, because she didn't want to "pass judgment"; she felt the mother was trying hard to be a better parent. In fact, protecting children from parental harm is no different from protecting them from an infection risk or a physical hazard like a busy street. A truly nonjudgmental physician can simultaneously intervene to protect children while striving to maintain a caring, engaged connection with distraught parents. The parents, out of anger, may not initially reciprocate, but the relationship can be invaluable to them in the long run. Not being judged for their failings as parents but supported as they figure out what to do next, enables them to turn to their child's doctor for guidance rather than finding their way alone.

Avoiding judgmentalism doesn't mean you won't initially feel anger toward a patient who has harmed someone else. What matters is whether you can begin to engage with them anyway, responding to whatever happens during the interaction in the present moment rather than to past behaviors you probably haven't witnessed. When a student responded judgmentally to a situation of an abuser and Simon challenged him, the student asked, "How can I not listen to what is in my heart?" Simon replied, "By remembering that everything that is in your heart is going through your brain." While judgmentalism is driven by a noncognitive, emotive response to another individual, it is only our rational mind that can intervene.

Judgmentalism is an insidious process working in the background to degrade many routine clinical interactions as well, even when a patient hasn't caused anyone harm. It seems particularly prevalent among physicians in response to obese patients. For an unannounced standardized patient study I was conducting, we hired several actors, one of whom just happened to be overweight. He had the frustrating experience of physicians focusing on his weight rather than listening and responding to whatever else he brought up as a part of his script. He said he felt badgered by many of them to the point of having trouble hiding his irritation. The physicians' judgmental attitude so preoccupied them that they were unable to provide effective care.

It's hard to say if physicians are more judgmental than other people. I do think physicians are particularly judgmental of themselves, which in turn shapes how they respond to others. We self-obsess over all sorts of things, as if that does any good. A rather judgmental medical student was chastising himself while confiding to Simon that he watched a lot of Internet pornography, prompting Simon to ask, "What do you think is wrong with that?" The student replied, "Well, it's sinful!" Simon said, "So you think you may be doing something wrong in the eyes of God?" "Yes," the student answered. Simon concluded, "Why don't you let God deal with it? If he's unhappy, he'll punish you." The student smiled and said "Thank you." The message implicit in the question was liberating: If you can't come up with any reason why your behavior is wrong except that it's sinful, then why beat yourself up over it?

Simon's point is that judging ourselves is as fruitless as judging others. God can judge us, according to certain religious tenets, and we may be judged in a court of law, but regardless of whether we feel that we or our patient is a bad or lazy person, we should focus instead on the consequences—if there are any—of specific behaviors and what we are going to do to address them.

What makes us judgmental? I think it is hubris, which may be particularly prevalent among those who have the good fortune of becoming physicians. To judge is to forget one is not God. Who are we to decide that someone could have done better despite the cards they were dealt? And just as we tend to overlook the misfortune that leads individuals to self-defeating lives, we may discount the luck that enabled us to succeed. Instead we chalk up our achievements to hard work, resilience, intelligence, and our great personalities. But where did those come from? Once again, we must acknowledge that we too didn't pick our great genes, the economic advantages and/or nurturing family, friends, or community that enabled us to make it this far. Some of us were successful against great odds, perhaps because of an unusually resilient genetic makeup or chance events that worked in our favor. Whatever the reasons, they weren't ones we got to choose.

Hence, giving up the belief that people fail in life because of their own self-inflicted behaviors without acknowledging that those behaviors are the product of factors beyond their control, also means giving up the belief that we are personally responsible for our own successes. It can be a painful trade-off but well worth it. It enables us to forgive ourselves and forgive our patients, so that we can relate to them with a sense of shared humanity, collectively swept along in the river of life. And when we see them stumble, rather than judging them, we can think, "There but for the grace of God go I."

Questions for Reflection and Discussion

1. Can you think of examples of judgmentalism affecting patient care, like the one described in which a physician called child protective services before finding out why the family missed just one of many appointments, risking separation of a child from struggling but caring parents?

2. Can you think of an example in which you didn't ask a question because you made an assumption about a patient's motivation (for example, that they are not taking their health care seriously) when, in fact, there may have been some impediment, such as cost or fear, that got in the way of their following the expected care plan?

3. If you were caring for a patient who you learned was a registered sex offender, how might that information affect the way you relate to them? What if you also saw a note in their chart indicating that they are "drug seeking"? Would you be predisposed to dislike them? If they had significant long-term health care needs, would they be at risk of getting less attention from you as their physician than you give to other patients? If so, what could you do to correct that deficiency in the consistency of the quality of your care? If you learned that they had been sexually and physically abused as a child themselves, would that change your perspective?

4. How do you react to the epigraph at the beginning of this chapter that, essentially, we are all doing the best we can with the cards we've been dealt? Do you agree? If not, what are your objections? What are the implications of your point of view for how you as a doctor might relate to and care for a patient who engages in self-destructive behaviors, including not following your evidence-based recommendations?

FIVE

Engaging with Boundary Clarity

Never forget that you defecate, micturate, and fornicate the same as your patients do.

SIMON AUSTER (OFTEN EXPRESSED WITH MORE COLORFUL, CRUDE WORD CHOICES)

ONE AFTERNOON, I was staffing the urgent care clinic at a Veterans Affairs hospital and walked into an exam room to see a man in his 60s who was concerned about a rash on his penis. He looked apprehensive as I entered. When I said my name was "Dr. Weiner" (pronounced "Wiener"), his expression turned incredulous, he glanced at my name tag—presumably to verify that what I was saying was true—and then burst out laughing. Although his reaction reminded me of teasing I endured as a child, I could see that here it was coming from a different place. This was unpremeditated. He wasn't trying to entertain an audience, although the intern accompanying me looked amused. Rather, his response to my name in the context of his medical complaint was a stress reliever. Realizing what was going on, I felt some pleasure at how my name had actually been therapeutic, and also laughed. It would be easy to talk with this guy. We clicked.

To engage is, literally, to connect, like two railway cars that are latched together. Once linked, they function as a single unit. For the connection to work, the two cars must have the same destination. Also, they should be at the same level above the track, or the latches won't intersect. One car can't be looming above the other. And, when they do connect, they should come together gently with a satisfying "click" rather than a jarring "clack." Once engaged, each is affected by the movement of the other, such that a tug is felt as a pull and vice versa.

When I am introduced to new patients, I expect to engage, and usually that's what happens. After flipping through notes, looking up labs, or hearing a resident's presentation, I get to meet the person, who may be lying on an exam table, sitting in a wheelchair, or waiting on a bench against a wall adjacent to the physician's desk. Sometimes they are alone, sometimes with family, close friends, or a caregiver. One thing I like about meeting patients is that the purpose of the interaction is clear. I'm not walking in there wondering why we are conversing, as I often do at social events or cocktail parties. The railway car analogy applies: we're going on the same journey, which is their journey. And we're going to be at the same level. Of course I have expertise, which is why they've sought me out, but it doesn't elevate me. In my own mind I think of my medical training as a tool kit that I carry. I dip into that kit as needed, but the interface with the patient is always me—Saul—not the algorithms, protocols, and technical language that can dazzle and confuse laypersons while putting me on a higher plane. Finally, as we do engage, I will take care that the contact is gentle and not bruising to them, as they are exposed and vulnerable.

My impression is that most patients are eager to engage—but don't expect it. What they expect is a detached professional interaction that feels safe, if a bit impersonal. They have come to talk with a stranger about their hemorrhoids, depression, nasal congestion, erectile dysfunction, chronic pain, or simply fears of some lurking condition. When telling a doctor about an intimate and embarrassing problem, they assume the physician has heard similar stories a thousand times before and will take it in stride. I care for older veterans who exude masculinity, and I'm still struck by how openly they talk with me about sexual problems or drop their trousers to show me a diaper they're wearing because of incontinence. Patients count on health care providers not to humiliate them by recoiling in surprise or laughing inappropriately, and I think the vast majority of physicians understand and meet that expectation.

But detached professionalism is not as good for patients or their doctors as engaged interaction, as it lacks the affirmation and partnering of minds that comes with real human connection. Nevertheless, it is a widely accepted communication style for collecting medical information inoffensively, having an orderly conversation to arrive at a care plan, and closing out a visit. Patients find it generally unobjectionable, and many physicians find it familiar, safe, and efficient. They evolve a style that is serviceable in nearly any clinical situation.

When the role of "professional" dominates medical encounters, however, they become scripted, which wears physicians down over time, even though they are the ones adopting the persona. It's tiresome putting on a facade all day. It's also less fulfilling not to open oneself to the experience of real connection. As a result, in contrast to other relationships, physicians often find that while relating to patients they are giving, but not getting back. They become prone to see their work as a labor, or sacrifice, and to view each encounter as one more job checked off a list, rather than as a satisfying interaction. As a result, they may be less attentive to patients than they could be, even regarding patient care as a burden—in contrast to the way they might feel helping a friend—which is a recipe for burnout.

I've heard physicians say that they don't have time to engage, particularly with the short, back-to-back visits that are so common in office-based practice. This comment gives me the impression that they are not describing engagement, or at least not as I understand it. Engaging is the surest way to maximize the value of the time spent with someone. Engaging isn't an additional task; it's a way of relating in which neither party is holding the other at a distance.

It's hard to describe an abstract concept like engagement in a way that leads to a shared understanding about what, exactly, it means. I intend it to mean something quite specific. For those who think visually, the difference between detached professionalism and engagement can be understood by diagramming what engagement looks like, starting first within the medical context. In figure 5.1, physician and patient each occupy a space that is circumscribed by a boundary that defines who they are—their values, beliefs, hopes, fears, preferences, even their physicality. The space within which they interact is also circumscribed by a boundary; one that encompasses the medical context, inclusive of

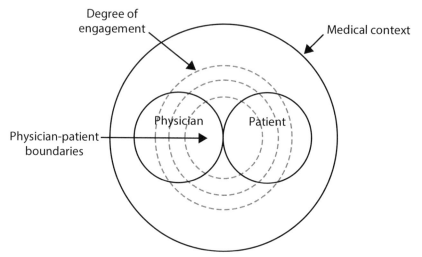

Figure 5.1. The role of boundary clarity and engagement in deepening the physician-patient relationship in the medical context.

the norms of the profession including all acceptable activities, whether "standard of care" or experimental, for which there is evidence of effectiveness or potential effectiveness.

Note that the boundaries of the two individuals are in contact, indicating that each of them is experiencing directly who the other one is. This is a natural state that occurs anytime two individuals are open to engagement. The dashed concentric circles illustrate how as the degree of engagement increases—for example, the extent to which there is a sharing of values and experience—more of the self of each individual is encompassed. As long as the interaction stays within the medical context, broadly speaking, increased engagement deepens the therapeutic relationship. Any interaction that falls outside the medical context, such as financial or romantic indiscretions, or renegade treatments that are unacceptable even when both parties consent to them would constitute a "professional boundary violation." Another type of harm, which is further discussed below, occurs when the physician encroaches on the patient's personal boundaries. Such intrusions, while remaining within the medical context, include badgering a patient for being overweight or pressuring them to have a procedure they feel uncomfort-

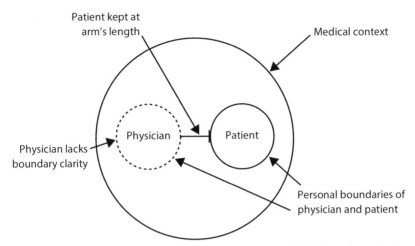

Figure 5.2. "Arm's length" care, in which a physician lacks boundary clarity and holds the patient at a distance.

able about. Such tactics, while potentially well intentioned, indicate that the physician is disregarding what may be going on inside the patient. Hence the physician must neither stray outside of the medical context, broadly defined, nor impinge on the patient's personal boundaries. This is not as hard as it sounds: If the physician remembers why they are there, can avoid being someone they are not, and has respect for the person who has come to them for help, they are ready to engage. If that person is able and ready to trust, the two spheres will naturally draw together and lightly touch, as if there is a small amount of gravitational pull.

In contrast to engaged interaction, detached professionalism can be visualized as a physician holding a patient at arm's length, as seen in figure 5.2. Note also that the boundaries of the physician are now shown as porous. This is to illustrate a physician who is not clear about who they are, at least in the medical context. My impression is that such a lack of clarity about self is the major reason physicians hold patients at a distance. Such physicians are hesitant to connect or are prone to withdraw at the slightest provocation because they simply aren't sure how to react to certain situations, so they adopt a persona. For instance, had I not been clear about personal boundaries, I might have appeared poker-faced or simply looked uncomfortable and vaguely offended in response to the patient laughing when he heard my name, a seemingly professional but aloof response. Fortunately, I recognized that a brief twinge of indignation I felt came from negative past experiences and that this patient's response to learning my name was a stress reliever, not a put-down. So I laughed along with him. The capacity to differentiate "what's me" from "what's you" is the essence of boundary clarity—of knowing who you are in a particular setting. If you don't have it, you feel vulnerable because you don't know what to think or do, which generates a sense of insecurity and defensiveness.

Boundary clarity is also what enables a physician to respond to suffering based on their patients' needs rather than their own discomfort. This was concisely captured in the satirical classic about becoming a doctor, *House of God*, in the dictum, "The patient is the one with the disease." It may sound harsh, but it's a useful reminder to the physician that what they are feeling reflects their internal response to what they are witnessing rather than what the patient is experiencing. While the physician must do whatever they can to alleviate a patient's suffering, getting caught up in that suffering as a consequence of a failure to recognize interpersonal boundaries will actually impair care. Thus, when a patient's sobs cause a physician personal discomfort, it is important for that physician to recognize that although the patient's distress is a result of the patient's situation, the doctor's own distress comes from within, an expression of their individuality, not the patient's suffering. It may be a caring response to the patient's distress; it may also reflect the physician's fears—fears of experiencing a similar hardship, of losing control, or of tarnishing the image they have of themselves. Or it may be a direct response to the recognition that the physician has unwittingly hurt the patient. Each of these situations calls for a different response—the first, an expression of sympathy; the second, self-reflection; the third, an apology.

Physicians who cannot make such distinctions generally hold patients at arm's length in the face of the suffering, rather than engaging. This was well illustrated in an essay in the *New England Journal of Medicine* by a mental health professional with a spinal cord injury who described how both a lack of boundary clarity and a lack of engagement by his physicians affected his care. He learned to withhold unpleasant information about his experiences with disability because their reactions were not helpful. He observed: "Expressing the emotions that accompany living with my disability evokes varied responses, but seldom has a physician responded by becoming more engaged or more determined to understand how my experience of disability can inform medical treatment." In essence, in an attempt to manage their own dysphoric responses to the patient's plight, his physicians kept a safe distance.

Boundary clarity is essential in interactions with patients who push boundaries, meaning they attempt to exert their will on the physician rather than share what they believe and seek what they want through respectful interaction. These are the patients whom physicians tend to identify as "difficult," sometimes labeling them as demanding, manipulative, seductive—terms often used to self-justify a physician's retreat from patients when they don't know how else to respond to them. Even as these interactions can provoke frustration, the physician who is clear about personal boundaries will remain open to engagement, respectfully asking questions to clarify why their patient is upset, unafraid of where the conversation may go. They will also provide fair warning about when the visit must end so that their patient can decide if this is how they want to spend the remaining time. Staying engaged is possible because the physician with boundary clarity doesn't take the patient's behavior personally and remains clear about their own values and priorities, and so is not offended or threatened if challenged. The patient, in turn, may find the physician's calm, unperturbed questioning and logic-based responses frustrating if they perceive the interaction as a power dynamic and are seeking to exercise control. However, it also provides them with an opportunity to begin to relate on healthy and constructive terms and hence has direct healing potential.

I've found that patients who try to push through boundaries respond in one of two ways when their physician is clear and firm about theirs: Either they stop the shenanigans and begin to interact openly and positively as they come to trust the physician, or they flee and find another doctor whom they can destabilize. The latter occurs if they are too distrustful to show who they really are, which is often a person frightened because they are unable to define their own boundaries and hence cannot let down their oppositional facade. In such instances, the physician will have lost a patient they probably could not have helped anyway.

There are rare situations in which a patient's challenging of boundaries should prompt even physicians with clear boundaries to intentionally disengage. These are instances in which the patient is not just pushing the physician's boundaries but is operating outside of the medical context, as when they exhibit physically threatening behavior or there is unequivocal evidence that they are seeking controlled substances for the purposes of diversion. I say "unequivocal" because I have seen too many patients suspected of such motives who were simply narcotic addicts, which is a problem within rather than outside of the medical context, and hence calls for a caring, engaged response.

As noted, harm to patients occurs when the physician is not respectful of a patient's boundaries. At the extreme, telling a patient that one finds them sexually attractive represents a total disregard for why they came to see you and, therefore, who they are. It is also outside of the medical context within which all clinical interactions must remain. The more common types of boundary violations can subtly contribute to the unintended infliction of shame or humiliation in the medical encounter, as in the example in chapter 4 of several physicians pestering a standardized patient about being overweight when he'd repeatedly indicated that he wanted to talk about another, unrelated, medical problem. For whatever reasons, they couldn't keep their preoccupation with his weight to themselves, which made him feel bad—even though he was just an undercover actor. Figure 5.3 illustrates such disruptions of a patient's boundaries, which occur within the clinical context.

As seen previously in figure 5.2, the physician's boundaries are again porous, indicating that, like the physician who holds patients at a distance, these "boundary-insensitive" doctors are also unable to reliably distinguish what's going on in their heads from what they are observing. They differ in that their lack of boundary clarity leads them to badger or pressure patients rather than to pull back. This occurs when

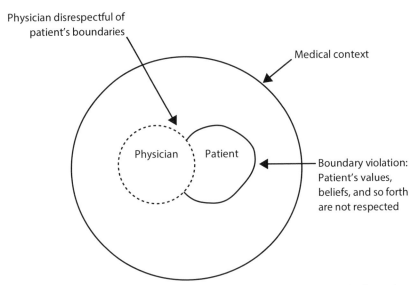

Figure 5.3. Intrusion on the patient's domain when a physician lacks boundary clarity in the medical context.

they feel strongly about something, such as their opinion that a patient needs to work harder at losing weight. They are not aware that their behavior is insensitive or even disrespectful. Because the underlying problem is a lack of boundary clarity, these are often the same physicians who hold patients at arm's length when they are not being patronizing or bossy.

Although the description above can give the impression that engaging with boundary clarity is very complicated, I think it is most helpful to think of it as a natural state. Engagement is simply what happens when two people are unselfconsciously interacting without a need to control the conversation in order to feel okay about themselves. This doesn't mean that they talk about anything on their minds. Engagement always occurs in a particular setting and context that both parties are mindful of. Engaging with a lover in a romantic restaurant or with a patient in an exam room are completely different scenarios, but within their respective parameters each is a real human connection. The boundary clarity that prevents an engaged interaction from becoming hurtful is assured when the two parties are respectful of each other, meaning that both refrain from trying to impose their wills, including their values or beliefs, on the other. Over time, this leads to increasing trust.

What makes engaging with boundary clarity so healing? In the immediate moment it is the affirmation. One afternoon when I was with Simon at the supermarket and the cashier asked her employer-mandated question, "How are you today?" He replied, "Do you really want to know?" She looked up, a little surprised, but when she saw that he was not being sarcastic or challenging—just asking a reasonable question— she replied, "Yes, I do." I don't recall what he told her, but Simon is almost always having a good day, and he briefly shared a few thoughts with her. She looked visibly pleased.

In the longer term, such sincerity leads to trust. Whether a customer at the checkout counter, friend, or physician, one comes to trust a person who is both open about who they are and respectful toward you, meaning that they don't pull rank on you, or attempt to exercise power, humiliate, or judge. You learn that if you look to them for advice, it won't be colored by any sort of agenda other than being helpful to you. This enables you to speak honestly, putting into words thoughts that you never fully articulated even to yourself, which initiates a process of positive change.

Consider a man who comes to the doctor every few weeks for help with managing several poorly controlled chronic conditions. He doesn't adhere to his medications because he is preoccupied with the chaos in his life. Relationships with his spouse, children, neighbors, and coworkers are distracting and volatile. The physician sometimes wonders whether they are doing any good for the patient but nevertheless welcomes him each time he comes to the office. Each visit they talk briefly but openly about what is going on in his life. He complains about various family members but rarely talks about himself. One day the physician asks him what he thinks he can do to help himself, since he can't make his family change. He acknowledges that he feels out of control in his own life and observes that skipping his medications is a symptom of "not having my act together." His doctor suggests referring him to a counselor, and he agrees that would be a good idea. Arriving at a place where he could talk about himself didn't happen right away but played out over several visits. His capacity to open up, listen, and accept help emerged out of an earned trust that his physician is a caring and nonjudgmental person who only wants the best for him. Unfortunately, physicians in training these days often have so little patient continuity that there are few opportunities to foster such therapeutic relationships even if they could do so.

How Do You Relate in Your Professional and Personal Spheres?

As we begin to participate in the medical workplace, we are taught to adopt a "professional demeanor." *Demeanor* is defined as a person's "outward manner." Is our demeanor consistent with who we are, or is it a persona? Whereas the former should not interfere with engagement, the latter will. A *persona*, defined as an "individual's facade or front" entails holding others at arm's length (figure 5.2) while giving the impression that one is not. In lieu of one's natural self, one substitutes a variant. It's useful to reflect on whether you adopt a persona and, if you do, what purpose it serves and whether you'd like to change.

Adopting a persona is, in fact, sensible in situations where engaging is demonstrably unwise. For instance, if you discover that the attending physician on your third-year clerkship rotation bases grades on how much they are flattered, I would recommend flattering them as long as you don't cross a line you are not comfortable crossing. You are in a situation where someone who lacks respect for boundaries is in a position of power over you, which is not a time to engage. Expecting you to meet their psychic needs is disrespectful of who you are, as a student enrolled in an educational program with career goals that depend on an objective assessment of your performance. Hold that person at arm's length while simultaneously pretending you are doing just the opposite. Adopt the persona.

On the other hand, as soon as rounds are over and you enter the room of one of your patients, you are now with a vulnerable person who needs human connection, no matter how grumpy or irritable they seem. Can you switch from portraying a persona to engaging within the medical context? And if the patient is emotional, whether they are expressing grief or anger, can you maintain clarity about your boundaries without pulling back? You may find the opportunity to talk with a real patient about their real life issues as a breath of fresh air after dealing with a high-maintenance supervisor. You get to be yourself again, and expend effort on an interaction that is meaningful.

Then, when you get home at the end of a long day, how do you relate to the people in your personal sphere? With your friends, do you engage and respect boundaries? What about your family? And, if you grew up with a parent who reminds you of your self-absorbed, boundary-violating attending, how has that shaped you? Are you wary of engaging generally? Do you end up in intimate relationships with boundary violators because their behavior, while disturbing, feels at least familiar? And when you get into conflicts with intimate partners, family, or friends, do your emotions compel you to lash out, perhaps disrespecting their boundaries? Or do they say that you are cold and hold them at a distance? Most of us have some of these issues, depending on the circumstances. Do you know what yours are?

The ideal is that we initially approach interactions with an openness to engage, a clarity about our boundaries, and a respect for the boundaries of others. This ideal applies equally to the personal and professional spheres. What you're engaging about, of course, greatly differs. As illustrated in figure 5.1, engagement in clinical interactions occurs exclusively within the medical context, whereas engagement in the personal sphere occurs outside that space. But that doesn't mean that you are any less you in the medical context than you are with your friends at a Saturday afternoon brunch (assuming you're not adopting a persona with them). The boundary issues in the professional and personal spheres are also more similar than different. With patients it entails knowing, for instance, not to nag them to do things they don't want to do even if you think they should, and responding based on reason rather than emotion when you feel they are giving you a hard time. So too with friends and loved ones!

In reflecting on your own capacity to engage and to do so with boundary clarity, a good place to start is with personal relationships, as those are where we first learn what we gain and lose by connecting with others and develop a pattern of response. Think first about when and with whom you engage positively. I'm referring to relationships in which you are open, are neither deferential nor patronizing, and don't have to tiptoe, meaning you can comfortably disagree without hurt or anger. That's possible because neither of you tries to impose views or beliefs on the other, indicating a mutual respect for personal boundaries.

Now think about what you are not prepared to share with these individuals, as a way of assessing how engaged those relationships really are (see "Degree of engagement" in figure 5.1). In college I was not prepared to disclose to close friends that I had a panic attack because I feared they would think less of me. Looking back, I don't recall any indication that they would have. An inability to trust close friends not to judge me cut off a resource that I could have turned to while feeling miserable. At the extreme, we hear of close family and friends who are shocked following a suicide, unaware of the pain the person had concealed. I think this is what the poet and writer Henry David Thoreau was referring to when he said, "The mass of men lead lives of quiet desperation."

Just as we may hold those who care about us at arm's length out of fear, we also, all too often, direct negative emotions toward them. If you find yourself succumbing to outbursts with intimates—be they parents, siblings, friends, or romantic partners—you may be blaming them for what you're feeling inside (a lack of clarity about one's own boundaries), or attempting to make them miserable too (a disrespect for their boundaries). These behaviors parallel those described in figures 5.2 and 5.3.

It's hard to say exactly why we have the relational issues that we do, but our parents, teachers, and peers in childhood have much to do with it. Collectively, during our most formative years, they create the only world we know. As illustrated in chapter 1, these early interactions have a lasting effect. I've had an easier time with boundary clarity in professional relationships than with immediate family. In my case, the challenges probably have their origins in the way adults and classmates related to me while I was growing up with a learning disability. Sometimes I respond with indignation to a benign comment from my wife or daughter that reminds me of things my mother or a teacher said when I was a child (for example, calling me irresponsible or lazy when I was actually just bewildered and confused) that led to insecurity and defensiveness. I've found that boundary clarity entails recognizing that the emotion I'm experiencing in response to an interaction often reflects my issues, not the other person's behavior. Recognizing that feelings—especially strong ones—need to be analyzed before acting on them is the biggest challenge to achieving boundary clarity in the personal sphere. Sharing with my family what I am feeling inside, but without implying they are responsible, is a way of engaging positively. It's something I've been learning and practicing.

Young adulthood is when most people struggle to define their boundaries, that is, to figure out their values and preferences. At such a vulnerable stage, what they need are people who they can safely bounce ideas off of, knowing that those individuals have their best interests at heart, and no other agenda. Many future physicians, however, grow up in families where their parents have a plan for them. It's hard to find your voice when people you are close to only want you to listen to theirs. Imagine trying to seek your father's advice about whether to become a doctor or pursue a career in music, when he has said for years that he expects you to become a physician or an engineer. The fact that he regards your career as something he chooses for you reflects a lack of boundary clarity. Lacking clarity about what are your decisions—not his—he may try to push you around in other ways too. You can't trust him as an unbiased sounding board who has only your interests at heart, although no doubt he thinks he does. Hence, you don't engage him in conversation regarding big decisions. Not being able to talk about your dreams and aspirations with someone who looms as large in your life as a parent can leave you questioning whether there is anyone you can trust.

If someone comes along, on the other hand, who you appreciate is an unbiased listener, it can be an eye-opening and healing experience. Not only is their feedback of practical value, but you learn that there are individuals who don't have an agenda other than to help. If you've not engaged with anyone like that before, it can be hard to recognize them even when they are standing in front of you. So, you may keep a distance. It's a vicious cycle, as you can only determine if someone is trustworthy by fully engaging and seeing what happens. Many people are absolutely trustworthy under most circumstances, but if you are incapable of trust, even those relationships will remain superficial.

Even if you don't have these issues, it's important to appreciate that many of your patients do. I meet patients who give off a vibe of suspicion as I enter the exam room. Others exhibit distrust more indirectly. They may seem agreeable with everything I've discussed for the care plan but then not follow through after they leave because they don't have confidence in what they've been told. How does one gain their trust?

Physicians who have good "bedside manner" can win trust in the short term simply by appearing trustworthy. Exuding reassuring confidence, they may convince patients to listen to them and do what they say even if the plan is not well thought out. But such a paternalistic style should not be confused with actual trustworthiness. Just like the physician dad who believes the best thing for his daughter is to become a physician even if her heart is not in it, physicians who believe they know best try to compel rather than to engage. Oftentimes I've heard a resident say a patient is "noncompliant" (which implies that a patient's job is to do as they are told) when in fact they are declining something they don't want, or simply are unable, to do. This reflects a lack of appreciation that the boundaries that delineate the patient incorporate both their individual preferences and their life situations. It also reflects a failure to recognize that the doctor works for the patient, not the other way around.

A trustworthy physician, in contrast, remembers that—like themselves—their patient is at the center of a complex life with many competing priorities that are all a part of who they are. Instead of trying to compel their patient to "comply" with anything, they'll respect those boundaries and seek a care plan their patient wants and can follow— one that is hopefully a step forward from whatever they are doing now. Rather than thinking of their patient as "not compliant," the trustworthy physician notes only that they are not adhering to a care plan, which calls for gaining the patient's perspective. They will find out, for instance, why their patient wants to leave the hospital before they are medically ready to do so, starting with the premise that they must have their reasons. Those reasons may be either shortsighted and misinformed or driven by competing priorities of great import. Either way, the physician will meet the patient where they are and respond honestly. They will not disengage because the patient seems to be imprudent in their choices.

In fact, it's at times when patients do the opposite of what you think is essential that they need you the most. I recall an Army veteran in his 30s with a serious bone infection that required intravenous antibiotics who insisted on leaving while he still had a fever "because I have to go pay some bills." The intern suspected the patient wanted to get high and told him he'd have to sign out against medical advice (AMA). To expect an addict to take your advice, however, and ignore intense cravings is not respectful of where they're coming from. This man had developed substance abuse problems after returning from two tours of duty in Afghanistan, where he experienced trauma. The fact that he felt a need to lie to us rather than just say, "Guys, I really need to get high," is an indication that we did not have his trust. What he needed most is a doctor who doesn't just give advice that he can't follow, but who cares about him. In this case that meant getting him oral antibiotics to take with him and encouraging him to come back as soon as those "bills" were paid. I think he knew that we knew what was going on and appreciated us for it, as he did return and was able to talk about his addiction during the readmission. We were able to get him into a drug treatment program.

When I was a resident and got paged that a patient wanted to leave AMA when we thought they were not ready to go home, I had them sign the paperwork. It always felt like a breakdown in the relationship between the patient and the care team that was, basically, the patient's "fault." Before they left, I'd explain all the reasons why they should stay, but I can't recall convincing anyone. Now I question the whole approach. The fact is, they have their reasons too, or they wouldn't be leaving. Heroin withdrawal, for instance, is a compelling reason to go get some heroin if you're the one in withdrawal. The fact that the patient has an addiction is just a part of who they are. As their physician, my job is to create a safe place where they can be open about it, so that we can work collaboratively in their best interest, whether to stay or go. From a medical-legal standpoint, I can document in the chart why they left and the extent to which I conveyed the risks. I can also explain what I did to mitigate the risks, like giving them Narcan, to reverse a possible overdose, to take with them.

The notion that success is actually about helping patients get the best possible care under the circumstances of their lives and preferences requires focusing on what makes them tick rather than on their not taking your sensible advice. When a patient declines a screening colonoscopy after learning how it can save them from a common and horrible cancer, the question is why they've made that decision, not how do I change their mind. Based on my research audio recording these discussions, many physicians either nag patients to get the test or stop bringing it up when a patient has said "no thanks" at previous annual checkups. A colleague of mine, however, recently described how after she had asked a patient annually why he didn't want the test, without receiving any satisfactory explanation for several years, he revealed that he had been sexually abused while living on a Native American reservation as a child. His wife was present at the visit and learned about what had happened at the same time as his physician. The man agreed to enter therapy for a history of sexual trauma, and a couple of years later the wife commented about how positively her husband and their marriage had changed. He also got a colonoscopy. This physician wasn't thinking of her patient as someone who didn't "comply" with her, but as an unsolved mystery that warranted continued exploration. It was not about her but about him. That's boundary clarity, and over time it led the man to trust her with a painful secret.

Perhaps the most contentious area these days where a lack of boundary clarity may undermine trust is opioid prescribing. Such lack of clarity can lead both to inappropriate prescribing and to withholding of opioids. On the one hand, a patient who is more likely to be harmed by than to benefit from escalating opioids may guilt-trip their physician into putting them on a higher dosage. The physician knows it's not a good idea but doesn't know how to assert that they are not personally comfortable escalating a treatment when the risks outweigh the benefits. In this situation the physician is allowing the patient to infringe on their boundaries.

On the other hand, physicians have also been forcibly weaning patients off of long-standing dosages of narcotics, causing havoc in the lives of individuals who were functioning well, when there is no evidence to support such action. There haven't been any studies to date showing that forced opioid reductions decrease morbidity or mortality, so this practice isn't evidence-based. Then why are physicians doing it? It's possible some are just misinformed. But it also may that they are reacting, unwittingly, to their own fears about getting in trouble rather than to a measured assessment of their patients' needs. Recently I saw a man who came into the urgent care clinic with his wife because chronic pain from an old back injury had flared since his doctor insisted at two prior visits on weaning a high narcotic dosage the patient had been taking for years. He worked as a forklift operator, never drank, didn't use recreational drugs, and had no history of obtaining narcotic prescriptions from anyone else. He supported his family and sent money back to parents in Mexico. The patient's wife vouched that he was missing work and at risk of losing his job. I restarted him on his original narcotic dose. Before writing the prescription, I ran the plan by the patient's physician, who was down the hallway, to confirm that I wasn't overlooking any information and that he did not object. I also documented how I'd concluded the benefits outweighed the risks.

I admit that increasing that dose of a potentially addictive pain medication made me uneasy. My unease, however, was not that I might be doing the wrong thing for the patient, but that I might get in trouble if there was a bad outcome. I've learned, however, that unease alone isn't sufficient reason not to respect a patient's wishes. One should not just react to what one is feeling inside without objectively looking at the situation. This patient had been functioning well, and now his quality of life and livelihood were compromised because of his doctor's unilateral decision. It appeared I could undo some of the harm with a stroke of the pen and protect myself legally by documenting my rationale in the medical record. I recognized that my unease wasn't related to anything the patient had said or done or any clinical research I knew of. It was probably the same unease that influenced previous doctors to pull the rug out from under this man. This was about them, not him.

I acknowledge that weaning patients off of narcotics without their consent can be attributed to factors other than a lack of boundary clarity. In some practice settings physicians are scrutinized or even penalized if their patients are on narcotics. Others may simply be ignorant of the lack of evidence, assuming that if starting patients on narcotics for chronic pain is bad, then getting them off narcotics must be good. A significant cause seems to be judgmentalism, as physicians often characterize patients who request narcotics as "drug seeking." All of these factors influence physicians' behavior. However, I do think we underestimate the extent to which we react to people, whether in the personal sphere or in our physician role, based on emotions that have little to do with the facts at hand. That represents a lack of boundary clarity, and it makes us less trustworthy.

Growing as a Healer

Your clinical skills are almost certain to grow during the course of your training and in the early years of your career. After taking care of hundreds and then thousands of patients, you will develop strong pattern recognition and reliable intuition about what actions to take, particularly when caring for patients who are very ill. But how do you grow as the person who is the physician acquiring these skills, so that those you care for benefit not only from your technical abilities but from who you are? Your well-being matters too: most people who choose medicine as a career indicate, often in their medical school applications, that they seek meaningful interactions with patients. And yet so many hold patients at arm's length, unaware of what they're doing. All they know is that their work is more depleting then fulfilling. How do you avoid this rut?

First, by not blaming your lack of connection with patients on "not enough time," the extensive use of technology in health care, or the electronic medical record. While I agree those are all problems, they are not the cause. Openly engaging with people is not conditional on anything. You can't chalk it up to being too busy.

Second—and this gets to the core—engaging with a diversity of people coming to you with a wide range of health needs requires attention to your own triggered emotions and how to interpret and respond to them. Self-awareness does not come easily, and the culture of medical training doesn't make it easier. Throughout your training and into your medical career you learn to suppress whatever you are feeling, whether it is fatigue, frustration, anxiety, or self-doubt, by adopting a matter-of-fact, even-keeled external demeanor. There is the sense that your medical career is happening to you rather than that it is in fact yours. The default is that over time you become an unobjectionable, technically competent task completer at risk for burnout.

To avoid this common pathway, you must acquire and maintain a perspective on what you are going through that requires balancing two realities. On the one hand you have, in fact, joined an all-consuming social system similar to the military, with conventions and expectations from peers and superiors about how to comport yourself moment to moment, and even what to think. On the other hand, you must remember what being a physician is all about: caring for people who are sick, worried about their health, or becoming increasingly dependent on health care as they age. Some are jerks, some are nice, some are lost, and some are confused—just like the doctors who care for them. There are reasons for their attitudes and capabilities, which you'll likely never know. They are wealthy, middle-income, and poor. They may look bored or indifferent, but they rarely are. They've come to see you, often at personal cost or inconvenience, because they trust that you are their best bet at getting the help they need.

When you are with a patient in a hospital or exam room, it's no longer about the medical tribe that you've joined; it's two people working together to solve the patient's problems. What do you feel as you walk into that room and start a conversation? Are you rushed, anxious, fearful, or frustrated that you don't have much you can offer, given the patient's condition? Impatient because of the circuitous answers to your questions? Burdened by responsibility? Distracted by other things you need to do, personal and professional? All of these feelings are common and normal, but they'll less likely distract you if you have one other: a desire to connect in some way, even if briefly. It's a natural state that you'll get to if you can strip away the impediments: pretensions, presumptions, insecurities, illusions, and anxieties that incline physicians to hold their patients at a distance.

Early on, my "physician-hood" consisted mostly of the skills and expertise that I acquired through education and clinical training. I often compartmentalized my interactions with patients from those with other people. Over time, however, there has been a significant shift in perspective. Now, when I walk into a patient's room, I'm reaching out to someone to form a connection. The "me" I'm introducing is inseparable from the one who can't cook but can wash dishes, can't find anything in grocery stores but enjoys the interactions with the stock clerks who help, and frets over every new ache and pain. Some may say that you can't get to this point until you are first comfortable with the technical aspects of being a doctor. I acknowledge that it's harder because, early in your training, you are prone to feel like an imposter. The best antidote, however, is to value the parts of yourself that predate your medical training and that can be such a comfort to your patients. You may still be "wet behind the ears" in terms of acquiring clinical skills, but at least you can give them the chance to interact with someone who—while still learning the basics—engages with them. There is nothing fake about that.

An openness to engaging isn't something you compartmentalize into your work or personal time, as it's your way of relating generally. I've found that neighbors, friends, colleagues, people in my wife's congregation, employees, and occasionally even bosses come looking for medical advice, often about sensitive, private matters. I take it as a sign that they regard me as approachable and safe. It usually starts with an e-mail or voicemail, or someone whom I vaguely know pulling me aside at a community event. I once had an employee call me from an emergency room because he was having a bad trip after smoking some marijuana and needed someone to calm him down. Just as remarkable as that call was the fact that there was nothing awkward about seeing each other the next day at work when he was back to his usual professional self. Just as patients are people, people can be patients. We are all in flux. When I got the flu and had a panic attack during a time my wife was abroad, I realized I would be comfortable calling many of the same people who had turned to me when they were in trouble.

If you can acknowledge your own humanity, you can more easily see others'. An indication that you are engaging is that you ask fundamental questions you otherwise might overlook or suppress. You see beyond what tests to order, pills to prescribe, or procedure to do, and notice the bigger picture. When I saw a patient recently in urgent care with a common cold who had survived two tours of duty as a soldier in Iraq and works as a data analyst, I asked him: "Is there something else on your mind, aside from a cold?" I learned that his PTSD symptoms were acting up, making him more anxious, and that someone he knew had gotten really sick from the flu, which triggered some feelings of panic. I recognized that the fact of his coming to see me was the real puzzler for me to sort out, not how to treat cold symptoms.

When I asked the resident who saw the man first why they hadn't asked the question, they replied that they had thought about it too, but didn't want to appear judgmental by inquiring why he bothered to come in. I wonder if they felt that way because it had not occurred to them that there may be some underlying reason other than just "worried well." Ironically, their fear of coming across as judgmental reflected that they were judgmental. If they'd given the guy a bit more credit—the same credit they'd probably accord their friends or themselves—they might have asked what was going on.

Medical training narrows your perspective about what matters during a clinical encounter. You're taught a lot of expert knowledge and reminded repeatedly, starting with multiple-choice testing, to apply that knowledge to patient care. So, when a patient comes in with upper respiratory symptoms, you focus on the symptoms, not on the person who has them. With such a narrow focus you don't form a human connection, and hence are likely to miss whatever is going on around those symptoms. A staggering 45 percent of people who commit suicide saw a primary care physician in the prior 30 days. I've come to appreciate that the safest way to be sure that I don't hurt my patients, and that I do help them, is by quickly forming connections so that I have every opportunity during the encounter to pick up on something I wouldn't want to miss.

And yet, when I'm observing physicians, all too often I see them holding patients at a distance. My research and quality improvement team, which listens to about a thousand audio-recorded visits a year, often has the same impression. What they notice most are the questions doctors don't ask when they hear patients say things like, "Doc, I'm *supposed to be* taking that medicine twice a day." It's not clear why they are not engaging, but my sense is that there are quite a few reasons, depending on the situation, including the following:

- They are task-focused rather than person-focused. In the example above, all they'd hear is that their patient is taking a medication twice a day, not the indicator that this is actually not happening. If it were their own child or parent instead, I posit that they'd ask, "What you do mean you are *supposed to?*"
- It hasn't occurred to them. For instance, when a patient has a cold, there isn't much to engage about, so it seems, so they focus on small talk while entering data into the computer.
- They don't know how. They hold everyone at a distance, including their families and spouses, unaware of what they're doing. They don't know what engaging is. This is likely due to a lack of clarity about personal boundaries.
- They've been taught by example to adopt a persona with patients rather than connect as who they are.
- They've learned that when they do engage with people, things can go sour fast. They are unaware that this is due either to a lack of clarity about who they are (that is, knowing what is inside versus outside the personal boundaries that define them at a point in time), or a lack of respect for other people's boundaries.
- They feel that engaging with patients is going to be draining,

consumes too much time, and isn't necessary. They are unaware that this perception reflects a misunderstanding of what it means to connect with people during even brief interactions.

- They would like to engage but are fearful of making themselves vulnerable.

Which of these, if any, apply to you? I think the last is a bigger factor than most physicians would acknowledge. A sign is that you withdraw in emotionally charged situations. When you're with a patient who starts to cry, can you sit there, aware that you are feeling all sorts of emotions—such as sadness, fear that what happened to them could happen to you, a sense of helplessness—yet remain calm and open, and not retreat into a persona? If the answer is no, I urge risk taking: avoid avoiding such situations. If you're experiencing emotions that pull you back in the face of suffering, instead let them wash over you—accepting that they are coming from within you, not from your patient—and remain open and in touch with yourself, perhaps by paying attention to your breathing. Also, be kind, thoughtful, and helpful to the person who is crying.

Physicians may retreat from the suffering they witness by focusing on medical facts so that they don't have to engage directly with the patient. I recall an extreme example when I took the place of another attending, supervising a team on the medical wards. The patient was a man in his 70s with emphysema so severe that he was kept alive with Bilevel Positive Airway Pressure (BiPap), a tightly sealed mask that forced air into his lungs with each breath. Even on the highest settings it was evident that he was gasping for air. It turned out he'd been in a miserable state for days and lung tests showed this was his new baseline. His present and future life looked like hell.

I asked the residents if they agreed with my assessment, and they nodded that they did. I asked if they had talked to the patient about withdrawing care, and learned that no one had. No one could tell me why. My conversation with the patient was straightforward. After introducing myself, I asked a few questions to be sure he was capable of understanding what I wanted to talk about. As the machine made whooshing sounds, forcing air in and out of his lungs, he nodded to each in a manner that indicated his mind was working fine. After explaining his medical situation, I asked him in about three different ways if he wanted us to remove the mask and put him on narcotics so that he would not feel air hunger but would soon die. Each time, without hesitation, he nodded "yes." We called his family, discussed the plan, arranged for them to come in right away, took him off the machine after putting him on a morphine drip, and allowed him to die peacefully within a few hours.

How long did these physicians in training, and their attending physician, watch this man suffer without meaningful hope of recovery? Why did they stand by rather than engage in what turned out not to be a particularly difficult conversation? I don't know for sure, but I suspect it was a response to fear of what they would feel by having this end-of-life discussion.

Regardless of the reason for not engaging, the remedy is the same: step outside your comfort zone. You needn't wait for extreme situations like the one illustrated above. In nearly every patient encounter there is an opportunity to connect within the medical context in a way that acknowledges our shared human experience. Start by looking at the epigraph to this chapter. Repeat it to yourself, replacing the medical jargon with visceral, crude language that strips away pretensions that any of us are other than flesh and blood with needs and desires. Let it sink in. Now you are ready to engage.

Questions for Reflection and Discussion

On Engagement

1. To what extent do you fully *engage* in various types of interactions, as the author describes the term? How many of your patient interactions are a boost to your mood or, at least, feel satisfying?

2. What parts of yourself do you show your patients, and what parts do you generally conceal? How might you behave differently when giving bad news to a friend (versus a patient) that your friend (or patient) has a serious illness or that a loved one has died? What

are the pros and cons of any differences in how you respond to friends and patients—for your patients and for you?

3. Do you feel your patients are benefiting from the distinct qualities that make you the unique person you are, or is that uniqueness not really a part of the way you relate to them? Do you feel you are interacting with patients in a manner that gives you a window into what makes each of them unique? Are many of your interactions rewarding? If so, in what ways?

4. If an adult patient came to see you with symptoms of a mild upper respiratory infection, missing work to do so for the third time in two years, would you wonder why they were seeking medical care, knowing that you just provide reassurance and over-the-counter medication recommendations for the common cold? What might be some underlying reasons for these visits? Would you ask? How might you frame the question?

5. Have you seen patient care situations in which difficult conversations were postponed at a cost to the patient's comfort or well-being because of a reluctance to engage? (The example of the patient with terminal end-stage emphysema kept alive on BiPap is an example.) If so, how might these situations have been approached differently so as to better serve the patient?

6. What are the implications of the epigraph at the start of this chapter for how to think about your patients' foibles, odors, and eccentricities? Can you think of a patient with whom you felt a strong sense of shared humanity? Can you think of patients who seemed "other" to you? What are the implications for how you interacted with each of them? Can you think of more engaged ways of interacting with patients who seem un-relatable?

On Boundary Clarity

1. When are you best able to be clear about boundaries, as the author describes the term, and when do they break down in your personal and professional interactions, leading to conflict, making assumptions about the other person, or distancing?

2. Are there certain types of patients who "get under your skin," making you cringe when you see their names on your appointment calendar? Consider what might be going on during your interactions with them, utilizing the framework described in this chapter. Is it that you can't engage with them? Do you struggle with maintaining boundaries when they make incessant demands? How might you alter your behavior so that these encounters become opportunities to model healthy interaction and to provide them a brief respite from the chaos that is likely present in their other relationships?

3. Have you ever felt resentment that a patient didn't show appreciation after you significantly helped them? If so, why do you think their show of gratitude is important to you? Does the doctor-patient relationship include an expectation that patients make their doctors feel good too? Could their indifference reduce your investment in their care? What if you learned from a patient's family member that the person actually does appreciate you but just isn't able to show it?

4. If a patient asked you a question about yourself that you were uncomfortable answering, how might you respond? Could it change the way you relate going forward? If so, how? Might you now hold them at more of a distance? If so, what—if any—are the implications for their care?

six

Caring

The most compelling way to show you care is to ask questions.

SIMON AUSTER

A LOT has been said about what doctors should feel. The Association of American Medical Colleges states that "physicians must be compassionate and empathic in caring for patients." *Compassion* is defined variously as "sympathetic pity and concern for the suffering of others" and as "sympathetic consciousness of others' distress together with a desire to alleviate it." No patient, however, has ever benefited from what their doctor was feeling—only from how they translated those feelings into some sort of action or interaction. I may feel terrible about your illness, but if I don't do anything to comfort you, how are you helped? And if I do act on those feelings with good intentions but without first finding out what you want, could I not make things worse?

What sort of physician emotions, then, facilitate effective care? Much has been written about the importance of *empathy* in patient care, an affective mental process described in Merriam-Webster's Unabridged Dictionary as "vicariously experiencing the feelings, thoughts, and experience of another." The term, which was first used in English in 1904 in an essay on art appreciation is the literal English equivalent of the German word *Einfuhlung*, which translates to "feeling into" a work of art. Empathy is often contrasted with *sympathy*. Whereas sympathy entails simply sharing the feelings of another, empathy entails sharing those feelings as a means of coming to an appreciation of the other.

Although there is disagreement regarding the exact definition, in a 2014 systematic review of studies to cultivate physician empathy, the authors conclude that "most constructions of empathy have in common . . . an understanding of the emotional states of others and expression of this understanding." Jodi Halpern, who has written a book about empathy, as noted in chapter 2, argues that the term has both cognitive and affective elements. These include "imagining how it feels to be in another person's situation," and "emotional attunement." Examples of the latter are "listening to an anxious friend, one becomes anxious" and "while talking with a coworker, one feels heavy, depressed feelings."

How do these feelings influence our behavior? Does the heavy, depressed feeling you experience in the company of a coworker, in Halpern's example, make you more or less inclined to reach out to them? If you do reach out, are your actions based on an accurate perception of what they need, or are they conflated with what you think you would want if you were in their situation? Might thinking you know what they need make you less inclined to ask? Without answers to such questions, how can one ascertain whether a physician's empathy is going to be good or bad for a patient?

In 2007, Simon and I published a paper arguing that the term *caring* is preferable to *empathy* for describing the ideal state of mind of a clinician healer, and we raised concerns about the latter in a section titled "The Trouble with Empathy." Now this distinction between two apparently similar words may seem like the ultimate "tempest in a teapot." Many think of the two words as essentially interchangeable. Why make a fuss about which one is better? We concluded that a lot is at stake. One of the challenges we faced was disagreement about the distinctions we drew between the terms. Some argued that we were just misunderstanding what *empathy* is, and attributing some of its positive characteristics to *caring*.

The purpose of this chapter, titled "Caring," is not to reengage that debate but to highlight attributes that are essential to a healer, attributes that I believe are better characterized by the term *caring* than by *empathy*. If some readers disagree about how I am using these terms and would say, "But you are describing empathy too," that should not get in the way of the aim here, which is to consider how feelings and thoughts can constructively—or not constructively—influence how we respond to others in distress or suffering.

To care is "to look after and provide for the needs of." Note that the definition specifies action, in contrast to *empathize*, which is experiencing a feeling. A recent story of a passerby who rescued a four-year-old boy dangling from a balcony vividly illustrates instinctive caring: Mamoudou Gassama, an illegal immigrant from Mali who had every reason to keep a low profile while strolling down a street in France, saw the child about to fall from the fourth floor. With athleticism fueled by adrenalin he scaled four stories and snatched the child from death, a feat captured by others on video. When interviewed about what motivated him, all he said was, "I like children, I would have hated to see him getting hurt in front of me. I ran and looked for solutions to save him and thank God I scaled the front of the building to the balcony." His response to the immediate need of someone in a precarious situation exemplifies caring as action. Others might have empathized with the plight of the boy, but that would not have kept him from falling.

Mr. Gassama's comment that he "looked for solutions to save [the boy]" illustrates the practicality of caring. Rather than drawing on what he was feeling inside as a guide, he looked at the situation analytically, asking himself, "What can I do to get to this kid quickly?" He then rapidly mapped a path up a vertical surface that he thought he could navigate and ascended from one outcropping to the next. Because he cared, all that mattered was finding a solution, whatever it would take.

Remarkable examples of caring do often happen in health care. They too are defined, however, by actions or gestures rather than by what someone might be feeling. In our essay, Simon and I described a perinatologist colleague who exhibits characteristics of an autistic spectrum disorder while exemplifying caring. His patients say that he rarely makes eye contact, staring instead at a notepad he uses to jot down what they say and then formulate questions. He doesn't touch them except to conduct a physical exam, not even shaking hands. Nevertheless, his patients rave about him, saying, "He always seems to know the right questions to ask to find out what is worrying me."

It also turns out that while he isn't good at making eye contact, he notices clues and pursues them. One day a Latina woman who didn't speak English came in for an exam, bringing along her five-year-old boy. The physician noticed that the child appeared hungry and got him a snack, even though he wasn't the patient. The boy turned to his mother and said something that the Spanish interpreter in the room translated as, "This tastes better than the rat we had for supper last night!" With more questions, the perinatologist learned that the family was living in an abandoned building and scavenging for food. In addition to setting up a social work consultation, he and the residents in the clinic contributed money, and a volunteer went out and bought food for them to take before they left. The perinatologist worked out a plan to get them a continuous supply of food until social services support could be implemented.

The physician behaviors that aided this mother and child consisted of observations, questions, and then thoughtful interventions based on the answers to those questions by someone who doesn't even make eye contact. In the way the term *empathy* is used in the literature, it would be hard to say that it was present here. Like the example of the man scaling a building, what we see is caring in action.

The case of Ms. G, described by Halpern and considered in chapter 2, of a woman who chose to forgo hemodialysis and die after her husband left her for another woman, illustrates the distinction between empathy and caring. On the one hand, Halpern considers how she might have taken "a more empathic" approach to addressing Ms. G's "conflict between talking and not talking, thinking and not thinking," presumably while reflecting empathically on what she may be feeling. On the other, Simon proposes openly expressing anger at the patient's passively allowing herself to be victimized—anger that comes naturally to those that care about her, such as her friends waiting outside her door. Seeing how all these people react, including her physician, may help Ms. G reframe her situation, transforming her from victim to potential victor.

Caring rarely requires such dramatic action; more often it is evident in small but purposeful behaviors. I spend part of my time in a VA clinic, where I supervise residents and often stay late to finish reviewing medical record notes. A couple of the attending physicians in adjacent offices make phone calls in the evenings to their patients after a long day, typically to discuss findings of test results or to check in on them. As many of the veterans at our facility are elderly and hard of hearing, I frequently overhear my colleagues speaking loudly into the phone. I'm struck that they don't seem to feel rushed to get off the calls. After explaining test results, they'll ask if the patient understands them and if he has any questions. Then, just when I expect them to hang up, they'll often ask if there is anything else the patient would like to talk about. From the tone of their voices it's evident that these are long-standing relationships. Their final open-ended question reminds me of a son or daughter ending a call with an elderly parent who lives alone. They just want to be sure everything is going to be all right. They care.

Asking questions is, in fact, the hallmark of caring. Not just rote questions, the kind one asks in order to fill in all the checkboxes or elements of a note in the electronic medical record, or those required to do a standard diagnostic workup. Those are sometimes necessary and usually required (often for billing purposes) but demonstrate attention only to the essentials of the job. The question-asking one typically hears when people care is a kind of probing that indicates they are really trying to figure out something about the person or their situation so they can help.

When we don't care that much, we tend to make assumptions rather than ask questions even when the stakes are high. Assuming someone is going to be okay rather than checking probably means one is not that invested in whether things actually turn out okay. On several occasions I've seen inpatient teams send a frail patient home from the hospital, assuming they have the social support and resources to get their strength back instead of finding out if that's really the case.

Disregarding clues that a patient is struggling also points to a lack of caring. As noted in chapter 5, the staff that listens to the thousands of audio recordings we collect of physician-patient encounters often comment in surprise at the questions that doctors *don't* ask. They'll say, for instance, "I just heard a case in which the patient's blood sugars have gone way up, and the doctor just added more insulin but didn't ask them what's going on," or "Listen to this one in which the patient said he'd been at home too ill to eat for two weeks and hasn't sought medical care, but the doctor never asks him why he didn't come sooner." On a lot of these audio recordings the physician seems preoccupied with entering data into the computer, based on their non sequiturs (for example, responding to "Doctor, it's been tough since I lost my job" with "Uh huh, do you have any allergies?"). It doesn't necessarily mean, however, that the electronic medical record is the only reason they aren't asking follow-up questions. If the computer were taken out of the room, they might still not ask about clues that their patients are struggling if they don't see it as their problem—if the sense of caring isn't there.

The Link between Caring and Engaging

What leads us to care? Why do we care for some people more than others? What is the relationship between caring, curiosity, and engagement? How does caring impact the way we feel about our work?

First, caring is not some saintly trait that only the most special among us express. It is a universal instinct found in social animals— including dolphins, elephants, and chimpanzees—as documented in numerous studies showing that they console each other after one is beaten in a fight, decline food if taking it would cause harm to another, and even assist injured members of other species. Dog owners know that their pets comfort them when they are distressed. A 2007 *New England Journal of Medicine* article describes a cat named Oscar who roams the hallways of a dementia unit and curls up with dying residents during their last hours.

Why, then, do some physicians exhibit a lack of caring, as when they don't respond to signs that a patient is struggling with a life challenge that may be impacting their care? I think it's because of a lack of engagement. It is as we form connections with others that we come to care about them. Our motivation for engaging, however, may depend on what we anticipate we'll receive in return. In our personal lives we may engage because the positive feedback and emotional support are often reciprocated. We may see fewer benefits to engaging in the professional setting of patient care.

There may be cultural norms, too, that diminish our motivation to engage in the professional sphere. Our society sanctifies the nuclear family: first find a "soul mate"; then have kids around whom life evolves. Politicians and other high-profile figures proudly assert that "my family always comes first" or, if they are fired, give as an explanation for why they are leaving the standard line: "I want to spend more time with my family." While "family comes first" may be a slogan, it sends a message about other relationships. And yet, becoming an engaged, caring physician really does require a broader perspective, akin to "It takes a village . . ." Otherwise one can have the impression that real connecting, engaging, and caring are only for family and close friends. That amounts to drawing a small circle around oneself that excludes people who happen to be patients. The result is a lack of engagement with the surrounding world.

The world feels safer and kinder when people come out of that cocoon. For over 15 years I've taken the same route to work each day and the same homeless man stands on a particular street corner where there is a long traffic light, either selling the newspaper *Streetwise* or simply begging. Occasionally people roll down their windows to chat with him, which he seems to appreciate as much as the money, as his face brightens up and he appears animated. They may have given him change on other mornings, but sometimes they just say hello. The conversations look relaxed, without expectation of transaction or evidence of awkwardness or pity.

Occasionally, I'm surprised by who cares about me. At work one afternoon, I was feeding patient documents into a shredder in view of the waiting room at the local VA where I work, and an elderly patient I'd never seen apparently got concerned about my fingers getting too close to the blades. He limped over to warn me that the protective safety shield was loose and that I should be more careful.

In medical training I've seen caring framed as sacrifice. A training module designed to teach residents about professionalism posed a scenario in which the family of a patient the physician knew well was asking him to come see her in the emergency room when the physician was about to leave the hospital for an anniversary dinner with his spouse. The "correct" answer was to delay leaving, in accordance with the imperative to "put patients first." Cases like this one, designed to illustrate putting patients' needs above one's own, pit the personal against the professional, in situations where the physician has to make a choice that seems to be almost a referendum on their character. On the one hand there is the symbolism of an anniversary dinner, which commemorates the most personal of relationships, and on the other hand the commitment to the profession—almost a marriage unto itself. Over the past 25 years there has been a gradual shift in expectations, from putting work first to "work-life balance." What hasn't changed, however, is the perception that work and personal life are a zero-sum game; that time invested in one is time taken away from the other. Work is often regarded as depleting and personal time as replenishing. According to American Medical Association surveys, average burnout rates range from 40 to 50 percent across all specialties, and prime coping mechanisms center around personal time: talking with family and close friends, and sleep. But what if the problem is a lack of engagement at work?

A major factor in burnout identified on surveys is depersonalization, which shows up as cynicism, complaining about patients and their problems, and devaluing others in the work sphere. In an essay on burnout in a Canadian medical journal, Karen Trollope-Kumar describes overhearing the following exchange among three physicians in the doctors' lounge:

I am sick and tired of the endless stream of complaining patients! Do they really value what I'm doing for them? Do they have any idea how hard I work?

You're complaining about patients—what about the government? What the hell do bureaucrats know about medical practice? I've got a whole raft of patients waiting for essential surgery. But how much OR time do I get? It's ridiculous!

On top of everything else, we have to take on medical students. The other day I had a real know-it-all who kept asking me if what I was doing was evidence-based. I'm really fed up!

What's missing from the litany of complaints is "too many bureaucratic tasks," which tops the list on US surveys but not Canadian ones, likely because the latter has a single-payer system that simplifies billing. Conversely, the second complaint—the one about waiting lists for patients—is not often heard in the United States because there are few caps on spending. The first and third, however, are not about system problems but about the state of mind of physicians. They reflect depersonalization: blaming patients and medical students for one's miseries. Depersonalization is the antithesis of engagement. People are no longer experienced as individuals, but as particular types of problems. Patients become ingrates and medical students, irritants.

With regard to the first complaint, that patients don't adequately appreciate their doctors: speaking personally, I've discovered that when I engage with a patient and then begin to care about them, any concerns about whether they appreciate me become superfluous. The moment a human connection is established I know they appreciate me as a person, because that is implicit in all positive, engaged interactions. For them to say, "Thank you very much, Doctor Weiner, you are so wonderful" is nice but unnecessary, and maybe even a bit awkward. On the other hand, to walk into the exam room and see their face light up when greeting me feels perfect. When that doesn't happen, there are other ways I feel satisfaction: With angry, self-absorbed patients I find gratification in indications that they are moving in a positive direction— and if they haven't changed yet but I've discovered a way to interact with them that may nudge them in a better direction and keeps them from getting under my skin, I feel accomplishment.

In sum, I've learned that if you care about your patients, you don't need or necessarily expect their appreciation. And the very idea that patient appreciation is owed to physicians raises questions about what the relationship is for. Expecting ego gratification from patients reflects a lack of clarity about the boundaries of the medical context (see figure 5.1). The patient has health needs, is often feeling miserable, and comes to you for help and relief. You are there to respond to those needs. To expect them to tend to your personal need for appreciation is asking them to interact with you outside of the medical context.

Finally, when the physician quoted above asked, "Do they have any idea how hard I work?," I'm left wondering whether some of that feeling of work burden comes from the effort of depersonalization itself. Engaging with patients is less work than holding them at a distance. For instance, when I'm open about my limitations—for example, that I'm not sure what's going on with them medically and would like to discuss the situation with another doctor—I free myself of the burden of portraying myself as all-knowing when I am not. Engaging with patients also feels less isolating, because they become partners in solving their health problems.

With regard to the third complaint: medical students who ask challenging questions. As someone who works with medical students all the time, I find this gripe depressing. The wide-eyed, not-yet-cynical interest of curious medical students excited that they finally get to care for patients is always refreshing. If they challenge me with a good question, and I don't have an answer, it's a win-win to ask them to go look it up and let me know what they find: I learn something new and relevant to my work without any effort, and they get experience finding answers themselves. When clinician educators react negatively to student curiosity and questioning, they are undermining the vitality of the next generation of physicians. Medical students need the support of their attendings in order to get good grades and letters of recommendation required to advance, particularly if they aspire to a highly competitive residency. So if they get negative vibes, they will rapidly adapt their behavior to expectations by hiding or suppressing their curiosity.

That's not to say that I find medical student education all fun. Students give endlessly long formal presentations of patients, often not proportional to the significance of the illness and without regard to the importance of particular symptoms. After listening for several minutes to a narrative that goes on and on, wondering what horrible disease I'm supposed to discern, I'll realize that they are telling me that the patient has a cold. I have to remind myself that it's a necessary part of the learning process. I suspect that the "fed-up" physician in the example above has no patience for student presentations and cuts them off after a few seconds. That was my experience as a student on a few occasions.

While these embittered doctors may come across as self-absorbed and entitled (to me they do!), it's important to appreciate that they seem to be in real pain. It's often hard to fathom that people who are earning good money, have high status, and are doing exactly what they set out to do are so unhappy. Burnout rates top 50 percent, and the suicide rate exceeds that of the population at large. Why are they miserable? I don't think it's for the reasons they give. It's doubtful they'd be contented if their medical students stopped asking questions or they didn't hear patients complain. They still wouldn't have what they need, which is something they aren't even aware is missing: human connection. They may not know what it is to engage, and they have little experience of caring about others with no strings attached.

It seems that many physicians exhibit a limited capacity to form human connections with others. Their detachment may reflect years of negative feedback when showing vulnerability, both during their upbringing and throughout the medical education process. They may have had little experience being nurtured by people who challenge and support them without expecting them to mirror their own image— that is, to conform. It's not surprising that many detach, undermining their effectiveness as physicians. One can become a competent technician, but not a healer, when the capacity to form therapeutic connections is impaired.

I use the term *impaired* to convey that engaging is not a skill but a natural way of relating when two people interact without pretense. The impairment is an inability to be open. An openness to engage is not the same as having good social skills. The perinatologist described above is awkward to the point of not even making eye contact. Yet he noticed that his patient's son looked hungry and got him a snack. As soon as he heard that the child's family was scavenging, he began to ask questions, which soon led to a series of actions including spending some of his own money to get them food. At no point does he adopt a persona. His social deficits are part of who he actually is, not a withdrawal from others. His intervention is highly personal and unconventional: responding like a kind neighbor, as he reaches into his wallet. He engages (for example, offers the boy a snack), and he cares (asks a lot of questions to figure out how he can help when he spots a problem).

While engaging seems to be the precursor to caring, not every act of caring is preceded by engagement. For instance, Gassama's rescue of the boy from a balcony was an impulsive act of caring, before which there was no opportunity to first engage. His stated motive for intervening was simply "I like children." I suspect he is someone who is open to engaging in a wide range of circumstances. While many people may say, "I like children," without meaning it, this guy showed he meant it! Individuals who don't retreat into personas naturally engage throughout their lives, which inclines them to become instinctively caring people.

Caring and Boundary Clarity

I don't think of myself as a particularly empathic person. When I walk into an exam room and see an elderly man in a wheelchair who looks disheveled and seems slightly confused, I don't imagine what it feels like to be in his situation, and I'm not attuned to experiencing his emotions. Rather, I get concerned about his home and social support situation. Does he live alone? Is anyone looking out for him? How does he shop, cook, and bathe? Has he fallen recently? Does he have an alert button he can use to call for help? As I listen to his answers, I'm also interested in how he responds, not just in the factual information he gives. How "with it" does he seem? If he is vague in his answers, I'll get more specific: for example, "Can you tell me what you had for dinner last night?" I ask all these questions because I would not be comfortable ending the visit without knowing whether he'll be okay. As far as I'm aware, that's all I feel.

In those occasional interactions where I may be empathic, it seems to backfire. When I've identified with a patient's pain—thought about what it must feel like—I've become preoccupied with what could happen to me! In particular, I see patients with chronic back pain, often accompanied by sciatica. Their suffering makes me think about how easily I could end up in their situation, to the point where I'm hesitant to lift even a suitcase and worry anytime I have minor discomfort in my lower back. I don't see how having those feelings makes me a better doctor. In fact, my tendency to resonate too much with these patients inclines me to ask fewer questions because their responses make me personally uncomfortable. Delving into all their daily agonies makes me squirm, so that I'm less open to engaging. That's a problem because it's important to assess the impact of their condition on their life, including work, having sex, or cooking—whichever apply. In addition, because I'm imagining what they must be feeling, I'm not thinking about the ways in which people can learn to adapt and cope with chronic pain. What's going through my head reflects my fears, not their reality. They may be developing coping mechanisms that I as their physician should know about and help them cultivate.

What I'm describing, in recounting my empathic response to patients with certain types of conditions, is not caring but a loss of boundary clarity. To deal with this response requires self-awareness that I have this tendency. I have to remind myself that my perception of their feelings is really about my anxieties, not their situation. Boundary clarity is knowing who you are: where you "end" and the other person "begins," as schematically illustrated in figure 5.1. If you have boundary clarity, you appreciate that the feelings inside your head are just yours. As soon as you believe you know what another person is experiencing based on your own feelings, you have lost that clarity. Thinking you know what the other person is feeling is an overestimation of one's capacities, a kind of arrogance. Even thinking that you know what a future "you" would feel were you to end up in the other person's situation reflects an unrealistic self-assessment of one's capabilities. All you can know is what you—and only you—are thinking and feeling in the present moment under a particular set of circumstances.

Such clarity points to just one option for learning about and helping others, which is asking them questions. If you have no illusions that you can feel their pain or know what it's like to walk in their shoes, you'll seek to find out by going directly to the source. The questions I pose, above, to the elderly man in a wheelchair stem from that sense of having no idea what's going on with him. As the conversation advances, I start to form a picture of his situation and whether I should and can do anything to help.

Some might ask, "If you can't empathize, then why would you care enough to try to help others in the first place?" I think caring follows from engaging. When you interact with someone with your boundaries touching theirs (figure 5.1), so that they are experiencing you and you are experiencing them, you naturally come to care about them. This is evident in the questions you ask, which reflect a genuine interest in figuring out what is going on rather than making assumptions.

Caring in the Clinical Setting

At the two medical centers where I see patients, many are at the bottom of the socioeconomic strata. Some live in shelters or on the street. It's struck me that I rarely engage with people experiencing homelessness who approach me on my way to work, but a few minutes later I welcome them in the urgent care clinic. They may not be the same people, but they have many of the same needs. Am I not the same person? The difference is that the second encounter occurs within rather than outside of the medical context (figure 5.1). I'm no longer trying to get to work on time, and the person coming toward me is no longer approaching me to ask for money.

Nevertheless, there is a risk that I will continue to hold them at arm's length. When someone at the bottom of the social ladder seeks care, the question arises whether their physician will be as open to engaging and, ultimately, to caring as they are for a well-dressed professional who looks like them. The research on implicit bias and discrimination in health care strongly suggests they will not. While studies don't specifically measure engagement or caring, they do compare both patients' self-reported experiences and objective measures of quality, which show significant differences based on race and wealth, among other patient characteristics.

When interacting with someone experiencing homelessness, the physician may be repelled by the sight of disheveled clothing, the smell of an unwashed body, or the manifestations of severe mental illness and/or substance abuse if present. If a patient smells bad enough, I am distracted from engaging with and ultimately caring as much about the individual. I wish I were more like nurses I've worked with who don't seem bothered by human stench or, if they are, don't let it get in the way of engaging with patients. I also have trouble when someone is especially hard to understand. Perhaps related to my learning disability, I seem to have more difficulty than most others in processing garbled speech, as occurs among many with very low levels of education or severe dental problems. Without an effective channel for communication, engagement is limited.

At the same time, it is extremely important. Just as with other patients who seem to be barely getting by, there are things I want to immediately find out: Where is this person spending days and nights if they don't have a home? Are they safe? Who do they have a relationship with, if anyone? Does our homeless veterans program know about them (if I'm at the VA that day)? Are they able to keep track of and take their medications? How did they manage to schedule this appointment and get here on the right day? As the conversation unfolds I notice how they communicate. Are they logical? Do they drift off on tangents? Do they seem anxious? As I formulate questions, I'm calibrating them based on what I hear. If the patient initially provides answers that are too vague, I get more specific, asking questions like, "What did you eat today?" and "Where did you sleep last night?"

I ask these questions to get a mental picture of the patient's life context so that I no longer feel as if I am working in the dark, so to speak. I've come to realize, however, that quite a few of the residents I work with don't seem aware that their patient even has a context. It's as if the person popped up as a multiple-choice question. When they present a patient to me who comes in for diabetes management, they'll rattle off a plan for ordering various labs and adjusting medications. When I question them, however, about the relevant backstory—what's going on in the patient's life that may be contributing to the poor diabetes control—they haven't any information. What crosses my mind at those moments is the question, "Don't you have an urge to know?" But I realize that in a busy clinic, an expectation of curiosity isn't convincing unless I can show how it matters.

If I sense we are missing relevant context, I'll follow the resident to the exam room and often uncover information that calls for a change in the original plan. At one recent urgent care visit I met an older man with poor diabetes control who had recently moved into a low-income assisted living facility, and it turned out that the transition had disrupted his routines. Among other things, he could no longer locate the calendar he used for keeping track of medications and appointments. We called his daughter, who was unaware of the mishap, and she agreed to get him a new calendar and help him back into a routine.

Later, when I asked the resident what she'd learned, the response was, "To figure out why he's not compliant, I guess." True, as far as it goes. But what she didn't consider was the following: how keeping a calendar indicates that this man has a determination to maintain order in his life, that his personhood has been disrupted by a major transition, and that he has an offspring ready to help but who needs help herself in order to understand what her father's needs are. These are strengths and opportunities we have to work with when caring for this man. And complimenting the patient on his resolve and his daughter on her readiness to step up will reinforce desirable behavior and show them that you are noticing—which is an indicator to them that you care.

Well-off, educated patients are less vulnerable in terms of lacking material resources, but they are still often frightened, confused, and emotionally distraught when a major acute or chronic illness sets in. And while doctors are more likely to take them seriously, they are also prone to another kind of bias, which is to assume "this patient is just like me." I often get that sense when listening to audio recordings from a project in which my research team sent mystery shoppers into suburban practices across New Jersey. Several actors were healthy, middle-aged people who portrayed upper-middle-class lifestyles. At a new visit by a male patient in his 50's, a male physician launched into a discussion about football, assuming his patient was a Giants or Jets fan, and carried on to a point that went beyond simple rapport-building. It sounded incongruous, given that we'd trained the actor to screen positive for depression and to decline a colonoscopy because his dad recently died of colon cancer despite having "seen doctors all his life." In real life he had no interest in professional sports. The physician was making assumptions rather than finding out what his patient was like. The actor went along with it the way people do when they are trying to seem interested but are not. While there was a lot of chat, they weren't engaged because the physician wasn't tuning in to whatever the patient might need to talk about.

When someone cares, they are less likely to make assumptions, because they don't want to take the chance that they might be wrong. Before chatting about football, a caring physician would find out what's on the patient's mind. That usually entails asking questions. This is especially easy to forget when we identify with a patient because they look like us. While there is a lot of emphasis in medical education on "cultural competence," which refers to the ability to interact effectively with people of different cultures, the fact is that we all are, functionally, living on our own planets. While I don't have anything against emphasizing cultural competence, I think it comes at the risk of forgetting how important it is not to make assumptions about those who apparently share our cultural identity. We are all unique in so many ways.

How does one go about discovering what's important in a patient's life that's relevant to their care? What is the thinking process? As both a primary care doctor and a health care researcher, I've found an interesting parallel between getting to know patients and getting to know complex social systems, such as communities, as they relate to a particular question or challenge. In qualitative research there is an approach to explaining how the social world works called "grounded theory." The aim is to arrive at a theory that is grounded in observations of whatever it is you are trying to explain. So, if you are trying to understand why certain minority groups are overrepresented among children referred for presumed attention-deficit/hyperactivity disorder (ADHD), you might observe and interview teachers, school administrators, parents, and clinicians until an explanation emerges that fits the data, refining your questions as you go along. I find this process analogous to trying to figure out what is going on in the life of a patient that is relevant to their health or health care. In either case, you don't know where your questions will lead. In fact, it's better not to have a hypothesis, but to keep your mind open. You are just trying to figure out what is going on.

A grounded theory approach stands in contrast to standard clinical reasoning, which is hypothesis-driven. For instance, if a patient comes to you with severe abdominal pain, you start with a relatively short list of possible causes and then, one by one, whittle the list down through a series of questions, physical exam maneuvers, and tests until you have a diagnosis. That's what we mean by "narrowing the differential." Whereas when someone has stopped taking their medications, you have to go into discovery mode rather than hypothesis-testing mode, because there is no list, meaning you don't even know what is in the realm of possibility, because every life is unique. Discovering, as described above, that a patient's poorly controlled diabetes was related to losing a calendar during a move to an assisted living facility and that the "treatment" was to engage his daughter to work with him and the staff required an open-ended approach to asking questions, followed by more questions, until it became clear what was going on and what to do about it. In the qualitative sciences this approach is called "constant comparison," and arriving at the point where asking more questions no longer yields additional useful information is called "saturation."

It may seem odd to call this process "caring" in the medical context, but I think that's exactly what it is. Rather than just making assumptions about why your patient isn't taking their medications, you seek to get to the bottom of the situation so that you can be sure you're helping them. It starts with asking open-ended questions, and as you come to appreciate the particulars, you plan next steps, building on whatever strengths and resources they already have. If that's not caring, then what is?

Questions for Reflection and Discussion

1. What are the differences, in your mind, between providing medical care that looks commendable based on a quality audit (for example, reviewing the physician's note and orders) and medical care that reflects a personal interest in your patient's well-being? Are they one and the same, or are there differences? If the latter, what do you see as differences? Can you give examples? How important do you think they are for a patient's long-term well-being?

2. Think about a patient whom you became personally invested in or really look forward to seeing. What about the relationship led you to care so much? Is it that they remind you of someone you already know, that they have a positive attitude, or that you feel comfortable being yourself around them? Try to be as specific as possible. Can you think of changes you could make in how you approach patient interactions that would increase the frequency of these caring relationships?

3. What are things you would want to know about a close friend in another city who has been discharged to home following a serious car accident and who lives alone? Would you be concerned about depression? PTSD? Whether your friend can manage without help? What questions might you ask to assess the situation to your satisfaction? Now suppose that you learned that a patient of yours was in a similar situation. How might your questions be similar or different?

4. What is the path that leads you to care about patients at a personal level? Does it start out as curiosity, prompting you to learn something about them that intrigues you? Does it occur with engagement and boundary clarity, meaning you interact without holding them at any sort of distance, but keep the relationship within the medical context?

SEVEN

Making Medical Decisions

Medical decision making can be described as answering one question: "What is the best next thing for *this* patient at *this* time?"

SIMON AUSTER

A LL PHYSICIANS who care for patients make medical decisions, sometimes dozens a day. And yet, as far as I am aware, hardly any of us have training in the process itself. I wish I'd learned in medical school that there are four types of information one should always consider: First, there's what you need to know to characterize a patient's *clinical state*, including their medical diagnoses, what treatments they're receiving, and how sick they are. This is the information you acquire by taking a medical history, doing a physical exam, looking at the medical record, ordering lab tests and other studies, and interpreting the results. The second is the *research evidence* for managing that clinical state, accessible in clinical decision support resources like UpToDate or federal websites with guidelines, and by looking directly at peer-reviewed journal articles.

The third, *patient preferences*, applies any time there are choices for evaluating or treating a medical condition that have differing implications for an individual's quality of life. Whereas physicians are best at knowing that treatment A is more effective than treatment B in a clinical trial, only patients can say which they'd prefer, depending on their particular circumstances and priorities. This is especially important when the stakes are high, such as whether to have surgery. However, the situation that comes up most frequently is how far to work up symptoms or findings that are probably not serious . . . but just might be. Physicians vary greatly in whether they "chase" things, just watch them, or do something in between. Patients are often not consulted about what they would like. When I staff the urgent care clinic, I see countless people coming in with little puzzles. They range from odd lumps, bumps, and rashes, to quirky pains, to unexpected findings on X-rays and CT scans and slightly abnormal lab values. My colleagues who work up everything reduce the risk of missing a serious condition but put the patient through discomfort, inconvenience, anxiety, and potential complications of the evaluation itself. My more laissez-faire approach spares patients those stressors but may increase the chance that something significant is missed or caught too late. Hence the decision about how aggressively to evaluate a condition should include input from patients. Typically, I tell patients why I'm inclined to watch something rather than refer them for further testing right away, and ask if they have any questions or concerns.

Reflecting on this approach, a first-year resident asked, "So, what if your patient wants you to order what you regard as unnecessary tests anyway? What if they have garden variety lower back pain and tell you they want an MRI to see if they have a tumor, and won't sleep because of anxiety until they find out?" My initial response to such a patient is to ask more questions to be sure I've not missed something that could indicate their concerns are warranted. If it becomes evident that I haven't, I'll share with them my clinical reasoning so that they can appreciate why I'm not worried. I'll also tell them about the risk of false positives: an MRI of any part of the body can expose "incidentalomas" that get everyone worried but are generally better off left undiscovered. Often they just need this bit of medical education to change their mind. If that doesn't help, I'll explore with them the source of their anxiety and try to address what I can: Might they have an undiagnosed mood disorder that needs treating, or know someone who seemed to have a similar presentation and did have a tumor? Finally, if none of that works, there are two remaining options: Order a "therapeutic MRI" on the grounds that while it's not diagnostically indicated and could even confuse the picture, it may provide peace of mind. I'll advise them that their insurance company may not approve the test, in which case they'll have to pay for it out of pocket. Alternatively, I could decline on the grounds that I am not personally comfortable ordering a study that isn't clinically indicated and might escalate their anxiety. I'll remind them that they can seek a second opinion. Which of the two paths I take is a judgment call. Fortunately, it is rare in my experience for a discussion about preferences to get stuck at a point where we can't reach agreement.

The fourth type of information is *patient context*, which, as discussed in prior chapters, refers to anything in patients' lives that is relevant to planning their care. In my experience, this is the one physicians forget about the most. And patients often don't speak up because they may not be aware that some aspect of their various life circumstances is important for the doctor to know about. For instance, someone who is taking a medication erratically because it costs too much may not know there are less expensive alternatives. Hence, physicians have to be on the lookout for signs—such as patients not refilling medications, missing appointments, or saying something like "Boy, it's been tough since I lost my job"—that might indicate the presence of a contextual issue affecting their care.

While these four types of information are all essential to clinical decision making, there are strong incentives for paying attention to the first two but not the third and fourth. You can spend your entire medical career mostly ignoring preferences and context while looking like a perfectly good doctor to anyone who audits your charts. Meanwhile, many of your patients are left miserable and unaware that their problems could be traced back to you. They'll rarely understand that there were reasonable alternatives to the painful surgery they agreed to, or that a less costly medication regimen for their diabetes than the one you selected could have kept them out of debt.

Take prostate cancer screening. My neighbor once asked me whether he should go along with his urologist's recommendation that he have a prostatectomy. His PSA had gone up, and a biopsy showed cancer, a word that frightened him. But not all prostate cancers are the same, and surgery can lead to incontinence and problems having sex. After I printed out a few papers and went over the data with him on patients with similar pathology findings—which indicated a low likelihood of spread—he decided to forgo treatment. Seventeen years later I still smile to myself with satisfaction when I see him out walking his dog, looking as healthy as ever.

It's easy to overlook patient preferences and context because health care quality measures focus almost exclusively on adherence to research evidence, which is also what counts in a court of law. But if the goal of medicine is to help people lead the lives they want to lead, they matter greatly. Cases discussed in earlier chapters illustrate the point. Consider Ms. Dawson, described in the introduction, who was referred to the preoperative testing clinic prior to bariatric surgery for obesity. Her *clinical state* was that she had a body mass index of 43.6, with complications of diabetes and hypertension. Conservative attempts to lose weight hadn't worked. The *research evidence* indicated that bariatric surgery could lead to long-term remission of diabetes, improved cardiovascular health, relief from depression, and less joint pain. Based on this information, she'd signed a consent form that also described the medical risks of the procedure.

However, eliciting *patient context* (by asking her about her son when she mentioned she was looking forward to the surgery so she could better take care of him) revealed that she was the sole caregiver for a young man with advanced muscular dystrophy who relied on her to bathe and feed him. Because she'd need an open rather than a laparoscopic procedure owing to a prior history of abdominal adhesions from gallbladder surgery, she wouldn't be able to safely lift him for over a month. Her surgeons probably weren't aware of the bind she'd be in, likely because they hadn't asked about her life situation.

When Ms. Dawson was asked if someone else could care for her son while she recovered, she said absolutely not. Personally tending to him was her highest priority—her *patient preference*. With all four types of information considered, going to the operating room looked like a terrible plan and, at Ms. Dawson's request, her surgery was indefinitely postponed. Had she had the surgery, she might have lifted her son anyway, risking opening up a surgical wound. One day she would likely benefit from bariatric surgery, but not then.

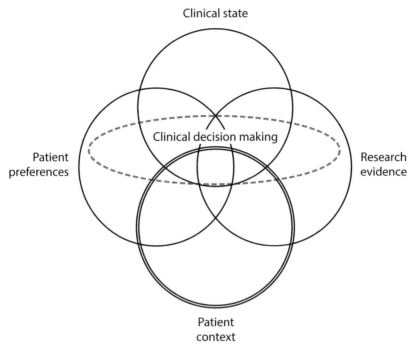

Figure 7.1. Clinical decision making should take into account and integrate the four types of information shown here.

Figure 7.1 illustrates, using a Venn diagram, how making clinical decisions entails integrating these four sources of information. I first came across it in 2004, a couple of years after it was published, but at the time it only had three rings. I wrote an editorial in the same journal illustrating the importance of including patient context and, years later, added a fourth ring to the diagram in *Listening for What Matters*.

My impression is that the major themes discussed in earlier chapters—problems with engaging, judgmentalism, and a lack of boundary clarity—all contribute to overlooking patient context and preferences. They result in a striking lack of caring. For instance, a patient requiring long-term anticoagulation was admitted to our hospital with an international normalized ratio (INR) of 9.0, an indication that he had somehow inadvertently ingested way too much warfarin (a blood thinner). He'd come in with a bleed in his shoulder joint, in a lot of pain. In the past, his INR was always between 2.0 and 3.0, where it should be. His doctors did all the right things technically, including giving vitamin K to reverse the effect of the medication and draining his shoulder. Remarkably, however, no one looked into why he had overdosed. Could he have early dementia that had progressed to a point where he could no longer take his medications safely? If so, is there someone to help him at home? Is his family even aware of what's happening? Does he have a pillbox? Is it time to switch to a different blood thinner that may not be as dangerous if you take too much, such as apixaban? No one asked these questions. The thought that comes to mind is: "Would you have overlooked them if this had been your grandpa?"

I think what happened is that the medical team just forgot the patient had a context. They were focused on the high INR and the swollen, tender shoulder but not much else. This elderly man existed in their minds only as a clinical problem. Social workers who could help were available, but only if someone from the team made contact and told them what the concerns were. Visiting nurses could go to the home, but only if someone put in an order to request their assistance. And there may have been family to help as well, if someone reached out to them.

In chapter 3, we saw a similar response when Ms. Garcia showed up repeatedly in the emergency department (ED) after missing dialysis. She got good care in terms of having her electrolytes corrected to prevent a lethal cardiac arrhythmia and, of course, she received dialysis. But no one asked her why she kept ending up in the same situation, so they didn't learn about her ill grandson whose health she prioritized. When that conundrum was finally uncovered, social workers got involved and moved her care to the same location as his, resolving the bind.

What all these missed opportunities share in common is that clues are overlooked, even when they are out in the open. An INR of 9.0, for instance, is a warning sign that a patient may be seriously confused or absent-minded. Yet from a strictly biomedical perspective, all the doctor thinks is, "Oh, I know what to do: this patient needs vitamin K." In the case of Ms. Garcia, the repeated emergency room visits for missed dialysis are a sign that she's overwhelmed for some reason. My research team calls these indicators that something might be going on in a person's life that is affecting their care "contextual red flags."

While doctors often miss clues about patient context, they are well conditioned to look for those related to a patient's clinical state. In fact, we have a hallowed tradition of labeling them, such as "Osler's nodes," "Janeway lesions," "Auspitz's sign," "Brushfield spots," or "Cushing's triad," each named after the doctor who first described them. The first two are clues that a patient has endocarditis; the third, psoriasis; the fourth, Down syndrome; and the last is an indicator of raised intracranial pressure. But what does showing up repeatedly in the emergency department because of missed dialysis signify? Or taking way too much warfarin all of a sudden? How about we call the statement "Boy, it's been tough since I lost my job!"—a clue that someone no longer has health insurance—Saul's sign? Doctors don't seem that interested in these contextual red flags. And I haven't seen any named after one. Yet the implications are just as significant for patient care. Context matters.

Why are we so inattentive to patient context? Largely, it's because we often don't engage. We actively hold patients at arm's length because we find their personal situations overwhelming. Our convoluted efforts are evident in the weird language we adopt when talking about them. A resident presented a 73-year-old "female" with colon cancer, who "failed chemo and radiation," "endorses" headaches, and "denies" symptoms of postradiation diarrhea. Why not simply describe her as a woman and say that she has headaches but not diarrhea? And patients are failed *by* chemotherapy and radiation, not the other way around. Our language often says more about us than about our patients. It reflects our need to keep a distance, and even to blame them for bad outcomes, rather than acknowledge our own limitations. Similarly, we don't pick up on passing comments like "Boy, it's been tough since I lost my job" when they engender feelings of helplessness, reminding us that we are not in control.

Second is the problem of judgmentalism, which is elaborated in chapter 4. Lecturing people about how they aren't taking care of themselves adequately presumes that they could do better if they had a better attitude. You'd have to think Ms. Garcia is pretty stupid and clueless, however, to think that she keeps coming to the ED because she doesn't know better. In *Listening for What Matters*, Alan Schwartz and I ascribed this reaction to the "fundamental attribution error," a social psychology term for the tendency to attribute other people's behavior to their personal characteristics while attributing one's own to situational factors: "If you screw up it's because of your laziness or bad attitude. If I screw up it's for reasons beyond my control."

Third is a lack of curiosity. This is tied closely to judgmentalism. If you think you already know why your patient keeps missing appointments, which is that they don't take their health care seriously, then why ask? When Ms. Garcia came into the ED repeatedly, the doctors weren't puzzled enough to ask her why. Their notes in her chart documenting that they'd told her how dangerous her behavior was indicated that they thought they already had the answer.

If we can stop being judgmental, allow our sense of curiosity to reemerge, and avoid convoluted language to keep patients at arm's length, we begin to ask commonsense questions: How did that INR get so high in the first place? Why does Ms. Garcia keep missing hemodialysis? We begin contextualizing care.

When you break it down into its components, contextualizing care is a three-step process: First, is seeing contextual red flags for what they are: clues to pursue rather than problems to shake your head over, sigh, and mostly ignore. The second is finding out what's going on. Start with an observation followed by an open-ended inquiry: "Ms. Garcia, I notice you've come back to the emergency room after missing your dialysis. Can you tell me what happened?" My research team refers to this step as "probing for context," which we listen for following each contextual red flag. It shows the doctor is paying attention to signs that a patient has a life issue that impacts their care and wants to get to the root cause.

Probing for context usually entails asking more than one question, which is why it requires curiosity. A curious person wants to get to the bottom of things. In the case of Ms. Garcia, that means going beyond knowing that she cares for a sick grandson to figuring out how, exactly, that has led to the ED visits. The aim is to understand enough to determine if anything can be done. The root cause of a contextual red flag is called a "contextual factor."

The third step to contextualizing care is addressing contextual factors in the care plan. For Ms. Garcia, that entailed moving her dialysis site to the same location as the clinic where her grandson received care. For Ms. Dawson, it entailed helping her think through the short-term implications for her family of her having bariatric surgery so that she could make a more informed decision. For the gentleman who came in with an INR of 9.0, there's no knowing what a contextualized care plan would look like, because no one probed for context. We don't know the underlying contextual factor.

While noticing contextual red flags, probing for contextual factors, and addressing them in the care plan are the three steps to contextualizing care, there are a couple of variations on this basic framework: First, probing for context doesn't always reveal a contextual factor that calls for a change in the care plan. When asked what's going on with her son, Ms. Dawson might have said, "He's going to have a baby!" Even though probing doesn't always turn up a problem to address, it's still good to ask, as you'll otherwise never know. Second, sometimes patients just tell you what the contextual factors are. If Ms. Garcia spoke English, she might have told the doctors in the ED why she was missing her dialysis. When patients reveal contextual factors without anyone on the health care team probing for context, they make it easier to contextualize care. Unfortunately, however, we've found in our research that doctors often still drop the ball. Even knowing why Ms. Garcia keeps coming back to the ED is no guarantee that her doctors will place an order for social work to address the problem. They may be too disengaged to hear what she is telling them. As discussed in earlier chapters, this problem has its roots in how doctors are trained and acculturated.

Whereas overlooking patient context reflects a failure to engage, disregarding preferences reflects a lack of boundary clarity. It's like going out to dinner with an acquaintance and ordering off the menu for them, assuming you know what they want. You've probably never done that because you know it's rude. In medicine, unfortunately, the habit is deeply ingrained. We are often oblivious to the line that separates research evidence from individual preferences. The surgeon who recommended a prostatectomy to my neighbor presumably understood the risks and benefits of the intervention. (I say "presumably" because specialists often see so many of the worst outcomes that they can lose their objectivity.) What he couldn't know without asking is what his patient would want if given unbiased options. Yet he said (according to my neighbor), "Mr. Davis, I recommend that we operate to take out the cancer. It may not spread anyway, but it's best to be safe." He also acknowledged that "there may be some side effects we should talk about." The problem is that he didn't elicit preferences. How could he recommend anything without knowing what his patient wants? Instead he might have said, "Mr. Davis, fortunately this cancer we've found may never harm you. Taking it out could cause some incontinence and affect your ability to have erections. Let's discuss the pros and cons. In fact, since there is no rush, here's something for you to read and think about. Let's meet in a couple of weeks and talk further."

Simon put it concisely when he said that medical decision making is figuring out what's "the best next thing for *this* patient at *this* time." The italics are important. The first "this" reminds us that each patient has a context and preferences; the second, that neither is static. Since you last saw a patient who needs help with activities of daily living, they may have lost a spouse who cared for them. Less momentous changes are more common and also need to be considered. Recently my research team recorded a visit in which a patient on a blood thinner described how he bruised himself after falling out of a La-Z-Boy recliner while dozing in front of the TV. Unfortunately, the footrest had broken and he'd tipped forward. The doctor was concerned about what to do. They came up with a plan for the patient to bring out an ottoman he kept in his bedroom so that he could put his feet up again. The doctor said he felt more comfortable about continuing the blood thinner. There is something poignant about such a mundane yet practical conversation. The physician's efforts to come up with a contextualized care plan through repeated questioning and problem solving exemplifies caring.

Eliciting patient context doesn't require getting a complete life history. Most things that happen in peoples' lives probably don't affect their health care. But when they do, they can be important. The three steps to contextualizing care save, on average, as much time as they consume during the medical encounter, according to hundreds of recordings we've analyzed based on the time stamps. The process is analogous to eliciting the clinical state: No doctor is expected to know everything going on in a patient's body; rather, we selectively pursue symptoms and signs until we have a diagnosis. Applying those same sleuthing skills more broadly, to elicit context and preferences before arriving at a medical decision, is the difference between a technician and a healer.

Questions for Reflection and Discussion

1. Think of a recent patient with contextual red flags such as a loss of control of their diabetes, frequently missed appointments, not refilling medications as expected, or showing up in the emergency department unnecessarily. What questions did you ask them, if any, to ascertain what might be going on? Were you able to get to the root cause (that is, identify "contextual factors")? If so, was there anything you could do to help?

2. Can you think of a recent contextual red flag that you didn't ask about? For instance, have you cared for patients who aren't following through on lab tests or referrals, or have declined a screening test or vaccination that you recommended, and not asked them why? Why do you think you reacted that way? Did you think there wasn't time, that you already knew the reason, or that there was probably not much you could do anyway?

3. Reflecting on the two examples above, where you did and then didn't look into patient circumstances that might account for behaviors that are complicating their care, are you comfortable with where you drew the line? Specifically, how do you decide when to better understand your patients' situations and priorities in the hope that doing so will lead to more effective care?

4. In chapter 5, a man with end-stage emphysema suffers from air hunger for days before he is given the choice to have his BiPap

removed and receive morphine so that he can die without further suffering. Can you think of examples in which patients you cared for were not given choices when they should have been? What lessons can you learn from those examples, and the ones presented in this chapter, about when to let patients know their options?

EIGHT

Healers Are Realists

Idealism often precedes burnout.

SIMON AUSTER

IN 1982, when I was in high school, I met a physician friend of Simon's who had worked at a Cambodian refugee camp, Khao I Dang, along the border with Thailand. It was a part of the world that was in chaos. First, the Khmer Rouge conquered the country in 1975 and brutally oppressed, starved, and executed millions of people. Then, in 1978, Vietnam invaded Cambodia to overthrow the Khmer Rouge. Physicians who worked with relief organizations treated patients suffering from starvation in settings lacking sanitation, with severe shortages of medicines and supplies, and few or no laboratory facilities. When monsoons hit, weak refugees drowned in their tents. Malaria was rampant. A large, international food aid program was established, along with a seed and fertilizer distribution program, which helped stabilize the crisis.

Simon's friend, Dr. Joe Julian, who was trained as both a neurologist and a physical medicine and rehabilitation specialist, recruited other health care professionals to work with him at Khao I Dang. I suspect that, as in Doctors Without Borders, they weren't paid much, so the decision to go was personal and values-based. I recall his observation that he saw a correlation between what they said at the interview and how long they stayed once they got to the camp. When he asked the question, "So, why do you want to go?" he heard a range of responses. On one end were those he described as "wanting to save the world." They talked in abstract terms about combating suffering and injustice. At the other end were those who responded in personal terms about what the experience would mean for them. They might say, "I think I'll learn something," or simply "I'll feel better about this horrible situation if I help." What he noticed is that those in the former category didn't last long. They expected things to go a particular way when they got there, which led to interpersonal conflicts, frustration, and burnout, whereas those on the "learn something" or "feel better" side of the spectrum just wanted to help. While also frustrated by limited resources and bureaucratic dysfunction, they sought to relieve the suffering they saw as practically and promptly as possible, rather than pursue a grandiose, unrealistic vision of saving thousands.

Dr. Julian's observation reminds me of the residency application essays I've seen from medical school students about wanting to travel to faraway places to fight poverty and disease. Then, gradually, reality sets in: they find that Medicare won't pay their residency stipend while they are overseas, so they have to use their vacation time or work without pay; or, they go on an international rotation, but no one tells them what to do when they get there, and they are mostly just sick with travelers' diarrhea; or everyone else is talking about doing a cardiology, or GI, or vascular surgery fellowship as the ultimate prize, for which working in a lab and publishing an abstract is critical to being competitive—not volunteering in an impoverished region; or they realize that few physician employers will hire someone who wants to take time off to go overseas because of the challenges of finding coverage; or their spouse is not interested, and they have young children to tend to now anyway. In the end, most drop the ideal of "saving the world" and end up in medical careers indistinguishable from those of their peers.

What these doctors and the ones who quickly left the refugee camps shared in common was that their expectations were not realistic. They underestimated what it would take to achieve the goals they had in mind and, as a result, overestimated their own commitment to pursuing them: "If this is what it takes . . . then never mind!"

There is, of course, nothing wrong with deciding you want a conventional medical career after exploring other options. If a medical school applicant who wrote about their dreams of working in Africa discovers that they hate the experience once they get there, and ends up a content and high-quality subspecialist in Scarsdale, New York, with a panel of patients who trust and depend on them, that is not a bad outcome. It's a perfectly fine outcome! They have found a setting in which they are comfortable engaging with patients, and they feel fulfilled. Research on burnout shows that such physicians are increasingly rare no matter where you look. No doubt they still experience annoyances, including patients who are demanding and entitled, and excessive documentation requirements, but they accept that those frustrations are just part of the package. They're realistic.

On the other hand, not all realists are healers. The burned-out physician who regards themselves as "just realistic" when talking about how medicine isn't fun anymore because patients are ungrateful, it's all paperwork, and the goal is to make enough money so you can retire young, is disengaged. They are stuck in a rut they don't know how to escape. In a literal sense, they are being realistic: if you can't form human connections, then the world is, in fact, pretty bleak.

Realists Can Do Anything

During my 11 years as director of a combined residency in internal medicine and pediatrics, I was struck that the residents whom I would most want as my doctor didn't start as adventurists trying to save the world; rather, they were practical people who liked to help others solve problems. And yet this groundedness didn't stop those so inclined from heading off the beaten path, embarking on careers that some of their peers wrote about in medical school applications but soon aborted. In fact, I'd argue, it enabled it.

For instance, Naina Bhalla, who has worked for Médecins Sans Frontières (MSF, aka Doctors Without Borders) for over a decade in challenging physical environments, didn't plan on an international medicine career. Her aspirations were unformed during residency. She seemed particularly concerned about patients who were dealt a bad hand, struggling with both poverty and illness. Many of the patients in our clinic came from impoverished communities. Naina considered primary care and infectious disease, which led to a couple of overseas rotations in developing countries. Based on those experiences, she gravitated toward international health, enrolling in and completing an international emergency medicine fellowship and a Master of Public Health degree concurrently after residency.

When she applied to work for MSF, the organization called me for a job reference that I've not forgotten because it was the most thorough vetting I'd ever witnessed. It sounded as if the group was trying to weed out the wide-eyed idealists and adventurists. Usually prospective employers for residency graduates called just to be sure there were no skeletons in the closet and to get a thumbs-up. MSF, however, had a trained human resources professional doing the assessments with the specific aim of figuring out if the person the organization was about to hire was the real deal or likely to crash and burn. In hindsight, I think the HR interviewer was doing the same work Dr. Julian did when he screened doctors who wanted to go to Cambodia. As MSF says on its website, working for the group is not simply seeking adventure: "By becoming a field worker you are acting in solidarity with populations in need." A sense of solidarity is an apt description of what I'd observed of Naina with her disadvantaged patients. She went on to work in war-torn areas in South Sudan, Ethiopia, Congo, Madagascar, Jordan and, most recently, in Rohingya refugee camps in Bangladesh.

When she headed off on her first assignment, in 2008, to a pediatric hospital in South Sudan, just west of Darfur, I asked her how she felt about it—in my own mind worrying about her safety. She replied that she feared that "I'll make a mistake and hurt a baby or child," and also commented, "I don't really think nine months is enough time for me to get to know a place the way I want to." She wasn't thinking about personal risk, but of what she might contribute and learn. While there, she periodically sent long e-mails to her friends when she could get access to the Internet. They conveyed both sadness and resolve, with a touch of irony and humor that showed she was okay. On Christmas she sent this:

> I wrote to Santa wishing for no death in the inpatient department; sad to say Santa did not grant my wish. The past few weeks have been difficult. I had about 10 the week of new years and 3 yesterday—sometimes I feel myself welling up with tears but know I cannot and try and wait until the end of the day and then it all sinks in and a profound sadness hits me. . . . I have had many babies die during my time here, newborns with neonatal tetanus, which is particularly devastating. The gut-wrenching thing is to know how easily preventable it is with just a vaccine during pregnancy. I have given each mother that came with a child a vaccine from our stock before leaving, although when their child dies in the ward it is sometimes hard to convince and explain to them why I am trying to give them treatment. I still think I may extend my time here if they need me to (as it seems they are having a difficult time trying to fill the existing positions here).

Along with sadness, she also found satisfaction, optimism, knowledge through experience, and even joy:

> I try and celebrate the small victories. I had 2 sets of twins which were premature and a bit less than 1 kg on admission who I was able to discharge, one on xmas eve, at each >2 kg. Both have returned for weight checks recently and are gaining weight and doing well. Also, I had a boy last weekend that had a proximal femur fracture who needed traction and had the logistician for the hospital help me construct a MacGyver-like skin traction set for him. He will be with me a long time (approximately 3 months), but overcoming these small obstacles sometimes is very rewarding. I even have had a few patients' families return to the ward with their child to simply show me they are still well, which is very nice. I am learning a lot, from the bad and good outcomes, and I am hoping, still trying to have at least one week of no deaths in the ward before I leave. Keep hope alive!

One also got the sense that she focused on the small things she could change that would make a difference. Here she describes some "home decorating" she was doing to make the children's ward more inviting:

> Anne and I are also on a mission to decorate the ward a bit, we bought
> blow up animals in the market (not really a whole lot of children's toys
> and such here) and strung them hanging from the ceiling in the ward.
> We are hoping to try and acquire some construction paper to make some
> more decorations in the ward and make it a bit more children friendly.
> I also found a bag of balloons which I use for therapy for the children
> who have been there for a while to try and get them up and about. It
> works fairly well although they very easily pop them and think I have
> a never-ending supply!

When asked about care packages by friends who wanted to send her
something to show their support, it was again the kids she was thinking about:

> I miss chocolate, cookies, pretzels, and good coffee; but really I am not
> missing anything immensely. Also, maybe some balloons or things for
> children in the ward would be great—maybe some crayons for the boy
> with the femur fracture that will be with me for 3 months.

What struck me as much as what Naina wrote about is what she didn't
say. Having worked for several months in Gabon, West Africa, and
studied health care in remote regions of Nepal, I know how frustrating
working in developing regions can be. Nothing happens the way you
think it is supposed to. On the one hand, there were the local staff,
who moved at a snail's pace even when there was a crisis like a child in
cardiac arrest. On the other there were the disgruntled, often imperious expatriates who were judgmental of the locals and wouldn't mingle with them. It was easy to become disillusioned. But if you held off
judgment, you'd start to understand things. For instance, that the nurse
who lumbered slowly toward you when you called for help because a
child wasn't breathing had learned from years of experience that that
child was going to die no matter what, and so she saved her energy in
the brutal heat for all the kids she'd need to care for that afternoon.

Pragmatists quietly soak up what's going on and figure out how best to move forward rather than becoming judgmental.

Pragmatists are also highly adaptive in their own lives, as exemplified by another former resident, John Scala, whom I first met nearly a decade before Naina headed off to Africa. John, who is tall, thin, and lanky, studied biomedical engineering at Johns Hopkins before attending medical school and then entering residency. Most people with that background head for the subspecialties rather than primary care. Circumstances and temperament pulled him in a different direction: John married a fellow resident in the pediatrics program who had come to the United States from Japan. Because she was on a J-1 visa, she was assigned to an underserved community, posted in Tooele, Utah, for three years. John made the most of the circumstances by building his own solo practice—literally from scratch. He actually designed and constructed much of the office himself, down to the electrical wiring. I wasn't surprised, remembering how he built our first website in the 1990s, well before resources like Wordpress or Squarespace had been invented. His medical practice became successful in a short time. Being in an underserved community with no one to help, John took call every night for four years.

Rather than hating or resenting his situation, John thrived. In hindsight, it's not surprising, as I recall what he was like during his training. What stood out for me when we met was not just his analytical mind, but how effortlessly he enjoyed his work and in what a low-key way. He was also especially helpful to others, especially when they were on call. This was before work duty hour limits had been set, so residents were often in the hospital late into the evening after having been up all night. They couldn't sign out until all of their patients were "tucked in" or discharged. It was not unusual for John, after he'd wrapped up his afternoon clinic and could go home (which is precious when you work more than a 100-hour week), to casually ask one of the post-call residents on a different inpatient medical service if they'd like any help finishing up care of their patients. I couldn't recall ever seeing anyone make this offer before, nor have I since. And yet it makes sense, if your mindset is simply to make the most of the situation you're in and help others.

After his stint in Tooele, John moved again to accommodate his wife's professional training requirements. They ended up in Coal City, Illinois, where he ran a practice for seven years, at which about half of his patients were uninsured or on Medicaid. He charged the former $50 if they were employed and $40 if they weren't, or "for free or for a couple cartons of eggs or some homemade cookies." A characteristic of people like John is that they take life one step at a time, learning as they go along. It's a given that the unexpected happens, and you just deal with it and move on. I recall that in those early years John and his wife were trying without success to conceive. One day he casually mentioned in an e-mail to me and another close colleague—in a mildly amused tone (like "whadya know?")—that he'd learned from a fertility workup that he has Klinefelter syndrome, meaning he carries an extra X chromosome. I mention this because I've found that people who are casually open about personal travails, and not too hard on themselves, are usually the same with others. They are safe. You know that if you share with them some personal misfortune or struggle they won't think differently of you either.

Missing the mountains, in 2011 John's family moved to Centennial, Colorado, a city with a population of about 100,000 about 14 miles south of Denver, where he started out working as a physician employee for a large health care corporation. After getting fed up with what he called the "layers of management, inefficiency, wastefulness, complete disregard for the patient, and greed," he set out solo again, opening Scala Medical. His doors are open to everyone, including Medicaid and self-pay patients, with substantial discounts for the latter posted on the website. He is also the referral source for young adults with cerebral palsy, Down syndrome, and other disabilities when they become too old to get their routine care from the local children's hospital.

Googling him now, 20 years into his career, I find dozens of glowing reviews by patients. A typical recent one describes him as engaged even when doing the ordinary:

Dr. Scala saw me for my yearly exam and then sent me for blood work. Cynically, my expectation was I would only hear from the doctor if there was bad news. Dr. Scala personally called with great news on my blood results, discussed my results in a way that I understood and his management plan for me and asked if I had additional questions. A very caring and compassionate doctor with a wonderful bedside manner in the "new medicine" where all of my friends complain about never having access to their doctor let alone being able to talk with him/her.

Dozens of people describe a caring guy who always has time to help out and gains people's confidence, like this one:

I saw him for a new blood clot in my leg. He knew I was scared and he took the time to understand what was important to me and what my specific concerns were. He listened to me. Even though he squeezed me in after his normal hours he wasn't rushed or hurried. I was very impressed by the thoroughness of his questions and examination. He was very reassuring and knowledgeable. He presented to me a number of treatment recommendations to manage my problem. I have a great deal of confidence in him. I was sent to him by a physician friend who is the Chief of Medicine at the Sky Ridge Hospital and she said he was the best. I agree and would recommend him and his partners to anyone needing a primary care physician. On top of all that I simply liked him. He was a genuinely nice person who seemed to genuinely care about my situation. His office staff was very pleasant and helpful too.

The physician these patients describe seems fully present in the moment when he is with each of them.

Folks like John remind me of the Serenity Prayer: "God, grant me the serenity to accept the things I cannot change, courage to change the things I can, and wisdom to know the difference." They are able to enjoy life because they don't get exercised about things they can't control, like not being fertile or getting posted for a few years to a remote location with no backup. Instead they expend their energy on finding solutions to achieving what they can *under the circumstances*. While many physicians dislike working as employees in a profit-driven, corporate culture, how many buck the trend by striking out on their own? I suspect the ones who do so, and are successful, are not so much adventurists as they are hard-nosed realists who work out a business plan, crunch the numbers, and after minimizing the risks through careful planning, give it a go.

Once they leap, they don't look back, freeing themselves to enjoy the ride, wherever it may lead. As a result, they are fully present to engage, so their days are spent in meaningful interaction, which is personally nourishing. Experiencing fulfillment through connection and enough financial success to meet their and their family's needs, they aren't motivated to chase wealth. That's something less contented people do. Not having a hidden agenda, like trying to get rich, they are habitually reliable. As a result, people trust them. Resourceful, caring folk like John bring stability to our communities. They give people hope and reassurance that the world sometimes works, and that there are people you can count on. That's part of what makes them healers.

Healers are also the most likely to succeed at tackling complex problems in their communities, because they not only care but are inherently practical in how they go about trying to make a difference. I saw such a grounded response in one former resident's approach to gun violence in her community: LaMenta Conway grew up in the Englewood neighborhood of Chicago, which is plagued by gangs and a lack of hope. She was the first in her family to go to college. She was also an accomplished gospel singer with the stage name "Sweetie," which follows her to this day. Her husband, Jacques, served as a pastor of the United Methodist Church by day while working as a police officer at night. When she enrolled in medical school she already had three young children—a three-year-old, a two-year-old, and a six-month-old. Her mother and grandmother helped with childcare. With their help, she graduated on time with excellent grades.

Over the course of her career in primary care, LaMenta has stayed closely in touch with her Englewood community through ties with extended family and the church her husband serves. On Mother's Day, 2014, she received a call that her 15-year-old cousin had been shot and killed on Chicago's far south side. Six months later, a 14-year-old cousin who had been an excellent student and promising athlete was paralyzed by a stray bullet. LaMenta had previously been involved in various mentoring initiatives, but these incidents prompted her to heavily invest her time and personal resources in founding the I Am Abel Foundation to "increase exposure, education and opportunities for underrepresented minorities . . . with a strong emphasis on developing a pipeline to careers in medicine." In an interview with her son, posted on the foundation's website, she says, "Violence exists where there is hopelessness," and that it is time to "reprogram the minds of city kids who have been told 'no' and 'you can't' and tell them 'not only are you *able* and capable, you are *Abel*, and yes, from the biblical story, you are expected to be your brother's keeper.'" Her biblical reference is to Cain's slaying of Abel in chapter 4 of Genesis. When asked by God where his brother had gone, Cain replied, "Am I my brother's keeper?"

Like Naina and John, LaMenta wasn't on any particular aspirational track during residency, but she was connected with her patients, who loved her. While the patients of the other residents in our clinic had an average no-show rate of 40 percent, not atypical when serving a low-income, urban community in those years when cell phones were still uncommon and people were hard to reach, LaMenta's patients nearly all showed up all the time. Given the prevalence in our clinic population of complex conditions such as diabetes, kidney failure, and chronic obstructive pulmonary disease, combined with poverty and a lack of social support, having some no-shows was a blessing, because visits tended to run over. LaMenta didn't get that luxury. No doubt her patients, who were mostly African American or Latinx (LaMenta also speaks Spanish), were drawn to this warm, motherly person who talked straight with them.

These characteristics are evident in her understanding of how to connect with the kids in her community, starting with the obstacles she experienced. In an interview posted on the foundation website, she says, "I and so many of my now successful colleagues were told by some incompetent student advisor what we could NOT do or accomplish. Thankfully, we had the strength to ignore the stupidity and irresponsible advice of those given charge over directing our futures and to believe in ourselves anyhow. I Am Abel Foundation seeks to empower, build self-esteem and help provide the building blocks of success." Second, she sends a strongly positive message about persevering and looking out for one another, referencing the foundation's name: "Our participants must recognize that because we are 'Able'—we are capable of amazing success and must accept nothing less. Because we are 'Abel,' we are also our brother's keeper and are each personally responsible for the success of our brother." Third, she writes about the compelling role of the church in her life growing up, without proselytizing: "The church was a community even for intellectuals. It was the place where movements begin and social activism fostered. It's where I found my mentors and where they told me 'Yes you can!' It was a place for the broken and broken-hearted. While drugs, poverty and despair were at our front door, the church was our refuge. . . . The church was also that place that if you had a talent, you would be discovered, because they would push you until they found out what you were good at!"

LaMenta speaks openly about her own missteps so students don't put her on a pedestal. She describes how she had no idea how to study or what was expected of her academically; how she got off to a rocky start and initially dug herself into an academic hole. She recalls how she was saved by a program for mentoring underrepresented minorities that got her on a track and led her to medical school with the skills to succeed.

The I Am Abel Foundation relies on many volunteers, mostly minority physicians and business leaders in the community, and a small, part-time staff. High school, college, and postbaccalaureate students are recruited from a variety of public schools in the Chicago area, with help from local teachers. A wide range of activities occur on weekends, in the evenings, and over summer break. The message, posted on the website, is that "it's important that you are not isolated. We are always better together. You need a village and we are here for you." LaMenta and her team continue to add new programs and activities, including Mental Health First Aid, intended to teach high school and college students how to assist those experiencing panic attacks, suicidal thoughts, acute psychosis, and other mood disorders—all of this while she continues to work full time.

LaMenta is candid when she talks about the stresses, reminding me of the proverbial duck who looks calm on the surface while paddling madly to stay afloat and keep moving. But the rewards are immense. She engages with young people who, instead of hanging out on the streets, are now excited about their futures as they learn first aid, CPR, how to take a medical history and to suture, and embark on trips with her and other volunteers to places like Cuba to learn about health care and resilience.

Realists as Healers

A characteristic that these three physicians, Naina, John, and LaMenta, share in common is that they focus on solving real-world problems, attending to what is going on around them rather than to some fantasy in their heads. They are realistic about the obstacles they face. Being realistic, however, doesn't stop them from pursuing their ideals. In fact, it enables them to.

Realists pick destinations that with sufficient effort are probably reachable, and then pursue them with tenacity. If, like John, your vision is building a primary care practice in a small community in America, but you aren't realistic, you won't understand that starting a business requires contending with local politics and onerous regulations, and establishing a network of relationships with people who will help you. Without realism, Naina could go on an international mission and quickly get fed up with the impediments that start as soon as the plane lands. Nothing works as it's supposed to: there's corruption and red tape; people move so slowly; getting anything done quickly is like trying to run in molasses. Those who thrive are able to sync with the local culture through real engagement and friendship, and without losing sight of what brought them there in the first place. Finally, if you start an organization like the I Am Abel Foundation to help address a need in your community, you can't expect everyone to rally around you at once and share your sense of mission. A professional fund-raiser once told me that benefactors support excellence rather than need. This makes it especially difficult to get off the ground with a charitable enterprise. It's hard to achieve excellence without adequate resources, but you won't get much support until people decide they're picking a winning horse.

Why do people like Naina, John, and LaMenta put up with all this? It's important to appreciate that their pursuit of an ideal is inherently self-interested, but in a good way. In other words, what they work hard at is not a sacrifice, but a labor of love. Rather than causing them to burn out, their work is a vital, positive part of their lives. That doesn't mean they love every moment of every day. Not at all. A lot of it sucks—the paperwork, the red tape, the fund-raising—but those are nuisances that don't fundamentally undermine the satisfaction and hope that they get from doing what they do. In addition, they stay connected with others throughout the journey. On a day-to-day basis, the sustenance comes through the relationships they have with others, as much as the small victories along the way.

The same can be said for individuals who don't venture off a traditional path but are fulfilled by their work. Recently I met a special education teacher who still loves what he does mid-career. He said he never expected to earn much money or get a lot respect. He learned early on that there would be long hours writing lesson plans, grading papers, and filling out forms. But he loves the kids and finds teaching rewarding and rejuvenating. When I asked him, "Who burns out?" he replied, "I think it's the ones who never really wanted to be teachers in the first place." Initially I was puzzled by his response because, after all, they must have wanted to teach if they entered the profession. But then I realized he was talking about engagement: teaching is about connecting with the next generation, one young heart and mind at a time. If you want that, then you want to teach. And if you have that, then the annoyances that come with the job are, well, just annoyances. They come with the territory. Accepting them is just being realistic.

Realists are also mindful of their own limitations, so even while outwardly focused on the well-being of others, they reflexively take care of themselves. They may not sleep quite enough or maintain the best diet all the time, but they are not into punishing or neglecting their physical or mental health. Self-neglect leads to skewed judgment. If you're in bad shape from not taking care of yourself, how are you going to have the presence of mind to observe and analyze other people's problems? To believe that you can is not realistic.

Healers are also realists who see the bad but don't let it blind them to the good. They may be pessimistic about the human race as a whole—seeing all the horrible things people do to each other, including war, theft, corruption, and subjugation—but quickly spot the spark of humanity in nearly everyone they connect with. This is in contrast to those who start out with high ideals but not a lot of patience for those they serve. They typically become disillusioned before accomplishing much. I see this with doctors who get fed up with their patients for not being "compliant" and appreciative. It's as if they like people in theory, but not in practice!

Finally, healers are also realists in that they recognize the world is a web of connections among individuals, and that they depend on that web. They operate within a social network, rather than trying to achieve goals on their own. They understand that the world really is a village, where personal relationships are everything. Their trustworthiness and caring put others in a good mood who, in turn, pass it on. They appreciate intuitively that while their actions may be insignificant in the scheme of things, they are not inconsequential. All great change starts locally, beginning with individual human interactions and then rippling out. An observation attributed to the anthropologist Margaret Mead encapsulates this truth: "Never doubt that a small group of thoughtful, committed citizens can change the world; indeed, it's the only thing that ever has."

Questions for Reflection and Discussion

1. What inspired you to pursue a career in medicine? Are you still inspired for the same reasons? If not, what have you learned about yourself or the profession that's changed your view?

2. Given what you know now, do you think you can have a career in medicine in which you find patient interaction rewarding and

meaningful much of the time? If yes, are you on course to experience those rewards, or do you need to make some changes? If the latter, what are you going to do to make those changes? Are you going to live with low expectations or look for something more rewarding?

3. Can you think of a physician whom you would be comforted to have as your doctor if you had a serious diagnosis that entailed extensive care with numerous uncertainties? If so, which of that person's characteristics appeal to you? Have you considered asking them what aspects of their work they find rewarding?

4. Are you concerned that you may experience burnout during your career? If so, what is it about practicing medicine or about yourself that is different from what you expected that accounts for this concern?

5. Do you have interactions with patients that are rewarding and meaningful? If so, are these rare or common? Can you think of a specific one? Was there something you did differently that made the encounter memorable? If so, can you think of ways you could modify how you practice and interact with other patients so that more of your interactions are as satisfying?

NINE

Physician or Technician? (Revisited)

Personal integrity means you make choices consistent with who you are, not just what you want.

SIMON AUSTER

A PEDIATRICIAN colleague has been complaining to me about a practice group he joined that seems to put productivity above quality of care. He described staffing their morning walk-in service all alone with no backup and seeing 15 patients, many of whom he didn't know, in a couple of hours. Not infrequently, he has 35–40 visits a day. He said there were times when he'd like to stop and make a phone call to another doctor, or look something up to see if he is current in his practice, but he'd fall behind. He recalled one woman bringing in her child the previous morning with a new diagnosis of ADHD made by staff at a local school. Looking sheepish, he said he didn't even glance at the forms before writing a prescription for methylphenidate. When he requested to see fewer patients, he was told that to do that he'd have to take a pay cut. His salary is currently in the sixtieth percentile for physicians in his specialty.

My colleague has to decide whether to see fewer patients at reduced pay, find a job somewhere else, or accept the status quo. For now, he's still with the practice and nothing has changed. He doesn't think he's harmed any patients, but it isn't the way he'd like to practice medicine. My perception is that quite a few doctors are in a similar situation.

What's the right thing to do? If you're unhappy in your job as a clinician, the first step is to figure out why. The example above is a particular kind of discontent—discomfort with the way one is compelled to care for patients. My colleague's concern was not with the impact of the working conditions on him, but on the children and families he sees. He didn't complain about all the notes he has to write during his lunch break or after clinic. While he isn't happy about the after-hours work, he understands that it comes with the territory. And while he doesn't find the practice management collegial, he can live with it. Finally, he's not too worried that he's going to make a catastrophic diagnostic error, given that most children are not that sick and he can tell when something is seriously wrong. No one has complained about his care, and he's passed all his quality assurance medical record reviews.

His discomfort is that he is not able to go below the surface with any of his patients. There's no time to ask questions beyond eliciting a symptom or asking about a side effect. Nor can he counsel patients and families beyond the most basic instructions, for example, "take this with meals." He enjoys the time he spends with patients, but there just isn't enough of it to get the job done the way he wants to. He feels that he is providing technically competent but not good care.

The problem of physicians functioning as technicians was introduced in chapter 1, "Physician or Technician?," but with an emphasis on the way doctors are socialized and trained rather than on time constraints. These are independent factors. On one hand, physicians with little interest in their patients as individuals aren't likely to change just because they have more time: they'll still elicit a perfunctory history and order tests, referrals, and medication changes based on this superficial information. On the other hand, those who really do want to figure out what their patients need are constrained if there is too little time to ask probing questions. Whereas chapter 1 focused on addressing the former, this chapter focuses on the latter.

However, while lack of time with patients is a real problem in health care in the current era, it's important for physicians not to let themselves off the hook too easily. We sometimes point the finger at "the system" while resisting looking at our own behavior. When I give grand rounds presentations on contextual errors, attendees often say they don't have enough time to find out what is really going on with their patients despite wanting to and knowing how. Two findings challenge this assertion, both based on research employing unannounced standardized patients (USPs). The first, mentioned earlier, is that in clinical encounters in which the physician successfully contextualizes care, the visit doesn't take longer than when others seeing the "same" patient don't. The second is that physicians often spend less time with patients than even the amount allotted. On audios we hear 10- to 15-minute encounters in 30-minute appointment slots for cases that we know are complex because we've scripted exactly what the actor will say and do. Once these doctors see on the intake form that their patient has, say, diabetes, and is new to the practice, they go on autopilot—punching in orders for labs and placing referrals for ophthalmology, podiatry, and endocrinology (if the patient has type 1 diabetes)—with little history taking or physical exam. They even finish their note during the visit, which entails mostly checking boxes or inserting boilerplate text. We see this often with one particular USP who portrays a young woman with diabetes who isn't taking her medication correctly. What doctors miss when they don't ask questions about the widely fluctuating blood sugars in the log book she hands them, is that she is depressed and has stopped taking her insulin whenever her new boyfriend is around because she is afraid of how he would react if he knew about her condition. Typically, they lecture her on the importance of being more compliant without first asking what's going on. The underlying problem for these physicians isn't a lack of scheduled time; it's that they aren't engaging, either because they don't know how or aren't interested. They appear just to want to get through the encounter fast. Their view of their work seems to be "I'll do my part, but it's up to the patient to do hers. That's not my problem." Hence the epigraph to chapter 1, which characterizes a technician as "one who knows every aspect of his job except its ultimate purpose and social consequences."

As discussed earlier, engaging with others is a way of relating in the moment and, hence, is not time-dependent. The preceding chapters have considered why many physicians don't engage, taking into account the milieu in which they were raised and the culture of the training environment. But an exploration of why they often function as technicians would be incomplete without also considering the circumstances under which they sometimes practice.

Specifically, even if an interaction is engaged, you still need time to examine your patient, discuss what you've learned, and arrive at a plan of care, which may require making phone calls, looking up information, reaching out to caregivers and so on, depending on the individual's needs. Many doctors who cut corners feel that it's because they don't have enough time to take these steps when needed.

If you are concerned that you are working under such conditions, as my pediatrician colleague is, I suggest that you first be sure you have diagnosed your situation correctly. In other words, are you engaging with your patients during the time you have? To accurately answer the question requires an awareness of what it means to engage and whether that is something you do. Consider the doctors in the diabetes example above who spent less than half the time allotted yet didn't even ask their patient why the blood sugar log she handed them showed sporadic periods of poor control. The audio reveals perfunctory interactions that are not engaged, such as their telling her that she needs to be more responsible with her self-care with no questions about what challenges she may be facing. When I debriefed them after sharing the data, many still maintained that the problem was a lack of time, despite the evidence that they were ending visits early.

If you are convinced, however, after an honest self-assessment, that you simply can't provide good care to your patients under your current work conditions, then the question is what to do. Fortunately, fully trained physicians have choices. Compared to nearly every other profession or occupation, they are in a seller's market—especially those marketing their skills in primary care. It is hard to overstate the job security of a primary care physician, given the nationwide shortage. Medical schools have been opening all over the country to increase the supply. As a residency program director, I saw how graduates were snatched up with aggressive recruiting tactics starting a year or more before they even finished their training. When one compares the situation to nearly any other occupation, the advantages are clear. Lawyers struggle to obtain jobs in the law even if they graduate from good schools. Architects, academics, and those trained in business have varying success depending on the prestige of their school, the region of the country they are in, and their prior experience. None match the consistency in obtaining employment in their fields enjoyed by physicians.

Hence, it seems hard to justify staying in a medical practice while providing what you regard as substandard care because of an unsatisfactory work environment. Most people in other professions have fewer options with comparable pay. Doctors can more readily up and leave. They are fortunate in another respect too: they earn a lot. The median annual salary of an American physician, according to Medscape Physician Compensation Report 2018, is $299,000. At the low end, family physicians earn $219,000, internists $230,000, and pediatricians $212,000. Young doctors entering the market often make more: In 2017, median starting salaries were $231,000 and $257,000 for family medicine and internal medicine, respectively. To put these numbers in perspective, consider that in 2017, a salary of $153,000 put you in the top 5 percent of earners in the United States and $300,000 in the top 1 percent, indicating that the lowest-earning specialties still land physicians in the top 3–4 percent.

When considering physician income, it's important to acknowledge that many start off with a lot of debt, averaging $200,000 with interest rates of about 5–6 percent in 2018. While that amount seems daunting, however, it's manageable when you put it in the context of what most people's lives are like. If one is willing to live at about the eightieth percentile for household income ($100,000 in 2017), after entering practice as a primary care physician and as the sole breadwinner in your home, you could likely pay off all debt plus interest in about two years. Of course, most opt to pay off the debt more gradually, enabling them to adopt the living standard of the top decile of earners right out of residency.

Given that doctors have such leverage in the marketplace, why do they stay in jobs when they don't think they are doing right by their patients? One explanation I've heard is that "it's bad everywhere." Physicians complain about the paperwork, hassles with insurance companies, lousy call schedules, pressure to see too many patients, and so on. But there are mitigating factors that make some environments better or worse than others. These include the number of patients doctors are expected to see, which is substantially driven by panel size (the number of patients assigned to them); how well they are supported by staff; the medical complexity of the patient population; the electronic medical record design; and receptivity of management to their input. Quite a few of my colleagues and former residents in full time practice really are content with their work setting.

Another explanation is that physicians, like nearly everyone else, are swayed by money. In other words, it's hard to trade a reduction in patient volume for lower pay, even if the pay—from the point of view of the rest of the American workforce—is still good. And it's easy to rationalize the decision. Few, if any, doctors will say to themselves, "I know seeing a patient every seven minutes is no way to provide good care, but I love the extra money." Instead they can say, "It's the system," "It's like this everywhere," "I've got to send my kids to college," and so on. These justifications work because each has merit. For instance, "the system" that runs health care is in fact pushing high volume in order to increase its profits. Its administrators have learned that many physicians will go along with it if they get a bit more pay.

Doctors are often not hard to buy off. When I was a resident and then a residency program director, pharmaceutical representatives swarmed the hallways of hospitals, clinics, and medical schools, pulling roller bags with one arm and carrying trays of food in the other. They were given free rein to open academic and educational events with a few words about their product, profoundly influencing American health care, the flow of money, and the integrity of science for the price of . . . a tray of brownies and some pizza or chicken wings. They also bore paperweights, tickets to sporting events, and other such perks—all giving them access to the inner sanctum where doctors write their prescriptions or learn about what to prescribe.

When I was in my final year of training, physician recruiters were invited to speak with us (also bringing food to noon conferences), about finding a practice position. They were paid on a contingency basis each time they placed a physician with a practice, so meeting us—all of whom were about to enter the job market—was worth a lot of pizza.

We, who were chronically exhausted yet hopeful about our futures, which could only be better than our current state, welcomed the respite. We could relax a bit, eat free food, and listen to a sincere-appearing, worldly, respectful, and usually attractive man or woman counsel us on what lay ahead.

One thing they all said was, "It's not just about the money. When you are looking for the right position, factor in quality of life, the environment, and the people you'll be working with." It was good advice (and in no way undermined their objective of convincing us to cast as wide a net as possible), but I found it hard to process at the time. Residency, which is mostly inpatient-based and supervised, is so different from private practice that it's hard to picture what you are getting into. One number that was easy to understand, however, was income. What I knew little about, however, was how a high salary is tied to productivity, which is measured in RVUs, or relative value units. These in turn are driven by seeing a lot of patients fast, and billing for as much as possible based on exhaustive documentation. I also didn't know how lacking in transparency the system would be. I'd be dependent on the bean counters living off of my productivity to tell me how productive I was. I wouldn't be able to independently verify what they said if they told me I needed to see more patients to earn my salary.

Once you've landed in a position and start to feel unhappy, it can be difficult to sort out what is going on. The reality is that you may have gotten there with a limited understanding of what's important to you, not as a resident, but for a lifetime career. A first step is to analyze your situation. The causes of physician discontent can be sorted into three categories: physicians' own characteristics, working conditions, and their perception of the quality of their care. As previously discussed, the first includes an inability to form meaningful connections with patients, such that daily work is not nourishing. In the second are all the hassle factors in the work environment related to clinical practice, including extensive charting, billing, ever-changing insurance company requirements, and dysfunctional management. The third applies when physicians see so many patients that they are not able to provide a level of care that they are personally comfortable with.

A lack of engagement with patients—the first category of discontent—is something physicians can't run from. Addressing it requires a new approach to interacting with patients, not going somewhere else. The latter two, in contrast, are both related to the practice environment, but it is important to distinguish between them because they have such different implications: Frustrating work conditions are so common that they are nearly universal. Most jobs involve hassle. One could even argue that the challenges of multitasking, doing a fair amount of pointless work, and dealing with imperious bosses are so universal that physicians should experience them just to know what their patients' lives are like. When work conditions, however, cross a line from personally irritating to the physician to precluding the ability to provide good care, they fall in the third category. They become a matter of conscience.

Where is the line between hassle and intractable obstacles to providing decent care? In other words, what is the difference between a practice environment in which you feel weighted down by tasks that soak up your time but don't fundamentally undermine your capacity to provide good care and one that leaves you uneasy that you are not doing right by your patients? I think it's a personal judgment call that is related to your ability to adapt to particular practice environments. In our book *Listening for What Matters*, Alan Schwartz and I wrote about a minority of physicians who were able to type away at the computer while remaining attentive to their patients, picking up on contextual red flags (like "Boy, it's been tough since I lost my job.") and probing them ("What do you mean? Tell me about that.") while most of their colleagues were distracted under the same conditions. Speaking personally, I know I am in the latter category. If I am listening to a patient, I am unable to put in orders or chart coherently, and vice versa. A workaround is writing parts of notes before and after a clinic and, when necessary, explaining to patients that I can't multitask and asking if they'd please sit quietly for a moment while I type or read something in their medical record. So far no one's seemed upset. As a physician practicing part-time in an academic setting, and most often with residents assisting, I have unusual flexibility. I have more discretionary time to catch up on tasks I couldn't do while in clinic. I couldn't provide good care if I were required to see five patients an hour on my own, without spending hours doing paperwork and note writing. When attending on a busy inpatient service for one-month blocks at a time, I've had to work every evening, before and after dinner, writing notes, checking lab tests, and billing. When I get depressed during those times, I remind myself that that's just the nature of the job combined with my limitations and other responsibilities. I'm burdened by hassle combined with my own slowness, but by doing extra work in the evenings I can provide what I consider to be acceptable care.

When unhappy in a job, I find the three categories described above to be a helpful framework for thinking about what to do next. Specifically, I ask: "How much of my discontent is due to a lack of engagement in the work? How much is my hating the chores that come with being a doctor in most practice settings? How much is that I'm forced to perform at a subpar level?" To answer these questions requires soul searching, as many of us give little serious consideration to the first, reactively concluding "It's not me!," and too readily pick the third over the second ("I'm being *forced* to provide shoddy care") when, in fact, we haven't made an all-out effort to find work-arounds and advocate for change. Each calls for a different response: the first entails figuring out how better to engage; the second involves seeking solutions and being realistic about the unavoidable hassles of modern work; and the third—living by our principles—may require taking a pay cut or moving to another practice.

Physicians underestimate the choices available to them. I suspect this is because the training process itself often makes us passive and accepting of hierarchy: Show up, work hard, and do what you're told. We soon become predictable, well-paid worker bees. Protective of our income at nearly all costs, we accept the status quo. We are risk-averse. But, as John Scala shows (in the previous chapter), we do have options, including striking out on our own, where we may be able to see fewer patients, earn equivalent salaries, and have control of our work environment. For those less adventurous, simply not holding ourselves hostage to maximizing income opens up opportunities to improve our working conditions. And, if quality of care is at stake, we have a moral imperative to do so.

When I was a junior faculty member, I attended a career development workshop for young academic physicians from all over the country where we talked about the circumstances under which one should leave a position. There was plenty of complaining all around as people described what they didn't like at their institutions: too few resources, not enough support, lack of collegiality, no respect for junior faculty, too much clinical time, lack of mentorship, and so on. I found the experience eye-opening, as I came to appreciate that what I was going through wasn't unique. In fact, it was typical.

The physician leader who was facilitating the discussion, Kenneth Shine, president of the Institute of Medicine (now called the National Academy of Medicine) at the time, observed that although it can be tempting to leave a position because the grass looks greener somewhere else, that is often not the best idea. Usually the time to leave is when you've made a positive difference and learned all you can, not when you are unhappy. Of course there are exceptions: one is that your principles are being compromised in some way that you can't rectify; another is that the place is toxic or hopelessly dysfunctional. Typically, however, a good time to move is when you've outgrown your current experience and are looking to develop professionally in ways that require a new setting and new opportunities. I've found this advice helpful when the question is whether to make a change. It offers perspective.

The message is either pessimistic or hopeful, depending on how you look at it. On the one hand, it's that you can't escape the real world, which is difficult, frustrating, and disappointing in many respects. On the other, if you can accept those realities and focus on your capacity to have an impact despite them, you'll grow increasingly resourceful, adaptable, and find ways to make a positive difference under nearly any circumstances. In deciding where to draw the line between "I can make the most of this" and "it's time to leave," you live by your principles, making choices consistent with who you are.

Questions for Reflection and Discussion

1. Have you found yourself in a situation in which you were responsible for others' well-being but did not have the resources, time, or knowledge to feel confident you could do the job well? (Having to care for too many patients in too little time is one example.) How did you cope?

2. If you've not been in such a situation, how would you know if you were? Imagine you were working in a busy clinical practice. How would you know that you were getting to the point where you were forced to provide a lower level of care than you'd like? What signs would you look for?

3. What might you do if you found yourself, like the pediatrician described, uncomfortable with the care you are able to provide given the number of patients assigned, and were told that you could see fewer at a lower salary? Under what circumstances might you be willing to take a pay cut? Have you ever been in a situation where you had to make a trade-off between what you felt was right and what would benefit you the most? If so, how did you respond?

4. Many, if not most, work environments have a fair amount of hassle, meaning you spend a good deal of time doing nuisance work and coping with difficult colleagues and bosses. These are manageable challenges, and they even provide an opportunity to learn to negotiate and adapt. Sometimes, however, workplaces become too dysfunctional to do your job effectively or facilitate meaningful change. They are beyond repair. Have you experienced either or both of these situations? How did you respond? What did you learn?

[TEN]

Healing as an Organizing Principle

Being a healer is not an identity; it's an organizing principle.

SIMON AUSTER

BECOMING A doctor was a big part of my identity well before I started medical school. I remember taking pride in the fact that I was a trained ambulance attendant and was going to become (I hoped) a physician. I saw myself as someone who would rush to the scene in a crisis and then know what to do. I dreamed about being an MD and knowing how to handle any situation when someone was sick. Becoming a doctor was a core part of how I saw myself and how I wanted others to see me. It felt a little as if I was going to have superpowers. No, it felt *very much* as if I was going to have superpowers.

I hungered to learn the secrets of the trade. It helped keep me going as I slogged through science courses, believing that at some point I'd be empowered. Early in my third year, I remember proudly meeting my parents at the front of the hospital wearing my white coat. I was in awe of senior residents, whom it seemed could casually handle any crisis they were called to respond to. Sometime in the middle of my second year of residency I too began to feel confidence in knowing what to do in most situations. If a patient spiked a fever, or become short of breath, or was overly agitated, or had dangerously abnormal labs, or went into cardiac arrest, I knew what to do. And with competence comes confidence. Not a bad kind of confidence—the good kind that enables you to stay calm so that you can think and intervene.

I now had the bona fides to back my identity as a physician. I not only wore the white coat, but I had the technical skills doctors are expected to have. What I had not yet figured out was that those technical skills are no more than a set of tools for me to draw on, when and if appropriate, when I enter a patient's room. One can spend an entire career never progressing beyond impersonally exercising technical expertise, and it's likely many physicians never do. But as noted in chapter 1, that makes you a technician, which is less than your patients generally need.

What they need, in addition to your technical competence, is your good judgment, informed by engaging with them and exercised while caring about them; in other words, they need you to be a healer. When patients are seriously ill or injured, the need intensifies, as their physical situation becomes profoundly intertwined with every other part of their lives. The feeling of being treated with indifference while in such a state can heighten fear, foster anger, and prompt what looks like irrational behavior.

A healer establishes a channel of communication that is wide and deep enough to allow for whatever needs to happen in the interaction to optimize medical care. In addition, their way of interacting is an antidote to the alienation many experience, sick or well. Specifically, it is that they relate with full and open engagement combined with a clear appreciation for personal boundaries, as elaborated in chapter 5. Unlike technical expertise, healing is not a set of skills but a way of responding to others. It is what Simon calls an "organizing principle." It does not come on and off with the white coat each day, as it is integral to who someone is. That does not mean it can't be acquired, a process that often requires letting go of the fears, doubts, and pretensions that lead us to keep others at a distance.

Why do so many doctors get stuck, developmentally, at the technical expertise stage, never exhibiting the characteristics of a healer? To begin to answer that question one must appreciate that being a healer is an aspect of the whole person. If the qualities are lacking in the personal sphere, they cannot be summoned in the professional sphere. Physicians who lack boundary clarity in the personal sphere, such that their interactions with intimates often veer into the volatile and unhealthy, are likely to be distant in professional relationships. This entails adopting a persona to conceal some of who they are. Unfortunately, the mask drops when they berate patients or staff for some slight. We periodically document these eruptions on concealed audio recordings our patients make for us of visits with their doctors. The patient will inadvertently say something that sets the doctor off, like suggesting a treatment plan the doctor doesn't like, and all of a sudden their voice rises as they get indignant or angry. The patient backs off, silenced and probably shaken.

These negative doctor-patient interactions are a strong indication that the medical training process has failed to cultivate healing as an organizing principle. If I had to name the dominant organizing principle for perhaps the majority of people going through the process it would be just getting through the overwhelming amount of work. It can be hard to value much else. Over time, medical students and young physicians become more cynical, depression rates go up, and disengagement sets in.

The obvious reason this occurs is that the training process itself is often degrading, as elaborated in chapter 3. Fundamentally, it does not reliably establish a safe environment for young people to learn to be comfortable with themselves so that they can enter into relationships with patients without having to adopt a persona. On top of that, however, the coping mechanisms young adults acquire in college and bring with them are often more escapist than nourishing. Escapist experiences distract you from negative feelings, including feelings of inadequacy, loneliness, and disengagement from others. Drinking, playing video games, and casual sex are generally escapist. Nourishing experiences promote a sense of well-being. Discovering that it feels good to stay home alone on a Saturday night with a good book and something nice to eat that you prepared yourself—that's nourishing.

Medical school felt, for me, more like a survival than a growth experience. In my first year I grappled with intense feelings of loneliness, not to resolve them, but to keep them sufficiently at bay so I could concentrate. I found solace in a couple of friendships with people I could confide in. A number of my classmates got together to hang out in small groups, play cards, and drink alcohol. They seemed to be having fun, but I don't know if those activities were more escapist or more nourishing. I tried a few times to join in but just felt more alone.

The medical education process seems to produce people with a strong identity as physicians but few who are healers. The inclination to connect with people, especially those who are anxious or suffering, is often missing. Early on a sense of personal accomplishment comes from the acquisition of new skills. Over time, however, as physicians become increasingly competent at the tasks of their jobs and medicine is no longer all-consuming, something else has to fill the void. Making lots of money, exerting power and control over subordinates, looking for recognition, and even sexual conquest are organizing principles for people in or outside of medicine who don't know how to engage. What they share in common is the desire for something more, whatever "more" is.

Not knowing how to engage, however, doesn't necessarily lead to materialistic or hedonistic pursuits. Most doctors just want to settle down with their families if they have them, take good care of their patients, keep up with the literature in their field, and find meaning in their work. But if their relationships are not positively engaged, something is missing. Over time, burnout sets in. Relations with patients and family may be similarly detached: they are workable, livable, acceptable, manageable, even at times enjoyable, but not nourishing. Increasingly they become irritants. The parallels between home and work are not an accident. An openness to engaging with boundary clarity is not compartmentalized. It reflects the way you approach most interactions. It's healing because it enables those you engage with to feel recognized and safe. And it is self-reinforcing because it feels worthwhile.

Healers work their magic in even the most mundane places. Recently I saw a young man engage some strangers in a small but remarkable way on a flight back to Chicago. The plane had landed, but they wouldn't let anyone off because the Jetway malfunctioned so there was no way to exit the aircraft. As time passed, several elderly passengers who appeared not to speak much English got increasingly anxious about missing a connecting international flight. Watching them become agitated, I thought, "Yeah, that really does suck. Glad I don't have a connecting flight!" I put my white noise headphones on and was about to resume reading a manuscript I was working on, when I noticed another passenger across the aisle starting to rustle out of his seat.

The man, who was in his twenties, tall and slim and wearing a t-shirt and flip-flops, leaned over toward them and asked where they were headed, communicating with gestures and speaking slowly while bending forward so they could understand him. He looked up their flights and confirmed the gates on his smart phone. He then pulled down each of their bags, and slipped backed to his seat. I noticed they were so preoccupied they barely acknowledged his assistance, but they calmed down. Perhaps it was because they now felt empowered about what to do. Once they were headed out of the plane, he grasped his own small backpack and followed casually down the Jetway, looking as if his mind was already off thinking about other things.

I was struck by his initiative to assist others, and in so natural and casual a way. He connected with them with a smile and touch, not in any official capacity but as a fellow passenger. I found the man's gesture heartening and likely a window into the kind of person he is. If he was someone who wanted to be a doctor, I'd consider what I saw a lot more meaningful than high MCAT scores!

Organizing principles are reflected in our behavior. We perceive them as a drive to do certain things, or simply as an unconscious response to particular situations. They show who we really are. This is in contrast to our espoused values, even our identities, which reflect what we believe about ourselves or would like others to believe about us. At this stage in my life, my dominant organizing principle seems to be work—mostly at my desk, mostly pursuing scholarly interests, including writing grant proposals and papers and, at the moment of course, this book. As to motives, I have no idea why. Do I want fame and glory? Am I seeking to do good work that helps others? Am I distracting myself from something? I don't know. And I'm not sure they are answerable questions. A more useful question may be: Is it fulfilling? If I got a fatal disease, would I have regrets about what I spent so much of my time doing?

Working at my desk is not the only thing that compels me. I am also compelled to engage with people—to close the distance that separates individuals and fosters aloneness and misunderstandings. As I'm cognizant that most people are not accustomed to engaging, I've learned to be careful about when to try to engage and to be aware of and attentive to boundaries when I do. I've found the best moments to engage are when others are open to engagement, which tends to happen when their equilibrium has been disrupted, such as by illness or the need to deal with something new or unexpected. People are often in that situation when they walk into the doctor's office. That makes practicing medicine a good fit for me.

When different organizing principles coexist in a single person, they can either compete or conflict. For instance, my writing competes with interpersonal engagement, since they can't both occur at the same time. But there is nothing contradictory about them. In contrast, organizing principles *conflict* when one directly undermines the other. It is not possible to be a healer who also swindles, bullies, or sexually harasses people. A healer is someone who respects boundaries consistently, not selectively. This mindset is incompatible with taking advantage of specific categories of individuals or causing them misery. On the other hand, there is no reason a healer couldn't acquire wealth by building a successful business that employs people, has a respectful culture, and provides a needed service.

Observing residents, I see the effect of a "just get through it all" organizing principle. Most are strikingly conscientious at their jobs. And yet they often narrowly define what that job is. For instance, while they are meticulous about prescribing the right dosage of the right drug for a particular medical condition, they are frequently oblivious to signs that the patient is too depressed, poor, or preoccupied with other priorities to take the medication as directed.

While they deliver a technically high level of service, it would be hard for me to say their behavior often reflects healing as an organizing principle. Their relationships with patients are typically too unengaged. In clinic, a resident might present to me a chronically ill patient who can't walk anymore, has trouble remembering their medications, or has lost much of their correctable vision. Depending on the situation I'll ask, "Do they live alone?," "How are they managing on their own?," "Who can they call if they need help?," and "Can they still use the stove?" Most often they don't know. It appears they are not seeing their patients as existing in a context but rather as tasks that fill their day. Finding out that one of their patients is homeless, and considering the implications for the rest of their care, doesn't much interest them. On the other hand, if I make a diagnosis they haven't considered, for example, saying, "I think those recurrent skin infections and sinus tracts are consistent with hidradenitis suppurativa," they're intrigued and look it up.

Some of the young doctors I interact with may have started out as healers. Like the young man on the plane, they might have been attentive to the struggles of those around them and responded unselfconsciously. But medical school can erode those characteristics. If I imagine the young man actually working his way through medical school, I wonder how he might change. After all-consuming years spent memorizing esoteric, disjointed facts he often doesn't understand, followed by endless numbers of multiple-choice tests and some bad grades, would he get depressed, inwardly focused, and distanced from the people around him? And, if he adapted to the new environment by learning how to be super-organized and disciplined, shutting out all that he used to notice, would the new way of life become a habit encouraged by good grades and other accolades?

As in medical school, when I was a resident, getting through each day was the dominant principle around which I organized my life. I focused on keeping up with numerous tasks—checking labs, ordering tests, answering pages, going on rounds with attending physicians, and admitting new patients—while not missing critical information that required immediate action. It took over a year, but I learned to be organized to the point where I had a system for tracking everything. I derived a sense of well-being from knowing I had this residency thing under control. I'd leave the hospital confident that my patients were "tucked in," even though I hardly knew them and had spent most of my time in front of a computer terminal or writing orders and notes.

In this environment, connecting with some patients some of the time remained a lifeline. Those encounters felt almost subversive, as if I was doing something I wasn't supposed to. I recall getting paged to meet with a family on a service I was covering one evening that had a litany of complaints about the care their mother was receiving, compounded by several failed attempts to get their concerns resolved after talking with the attending. After listening to them, I concluded they were right and told them so. I even enumerated for them my understanding of all the ways they had been mistreated. It occurred to me that unconditionally taking their side was unorthodox and risked solidifying their anger at their care team as I validated it. I wondered what the implications were for me of taking their side over "our side," imagining them telling the attending the next morning that I—a puny intern—had agreed that they were getting terrible care! However, they just nodded affirmatively and calmed down. I told them I was sorry about the things that had happened and talked through next steps for addressing each of their grievances, including how to file a complaint.

What occurred next was surprising and unexpected. As their anger at the hospital subsided, the tensions among them started to come out. They no longer needed to show a united front and looked to me to help them sort out some issues. Their individual personalities and the interpersonal dynamics emerged. I pointed out some pros and cons of their different opinions so as not to take sides and to model reasoned discussion, which seemed to work. By the time I left, after nearly 45 minutes, they were absorbed in talking with each other in a respectful way, having gotten over what they'd called me about. A couple of them gave a casual wave as I slipped out of the family meeting room almost unnoticed.

This interaction and others like it stick in my mind because they affirmed a fundamental part of me that was suppressed by the unrelenting demands of task completion, including writing orders, notes, and prescriptions, responding to my pager, doing procedures, and so forth. During these memorable encounters I wasn't working for a hospital, or performing for a residency program, or assuming a role to protect myself. Rather, it was me bumping up directly against the people I was serving. It wasn't a careless me, however. When I entered a room of angry family members whom I'd never met, whose loved one was desperately ill, I knew that I was walking into an atmosphere of volatility and complexity that required a heightened awareness of my boundaries and theirs. The decision to be myself rather than to adopt a scripted persona increased the danger of saying something wrong, but it also increased the reward. In contrast, a scripted persona would keep me allied with the institution, so that nothing I said could get me in trouble. But it could not begin the healing process for that family.

I wonder how many residents experience those moments of connection with patients and families that reminded me of who I was during my years of training. Had I not had them, I would have emerged a master task completer who can "work up" any patient and "manage" them, all with a refined doctor persona but little inclination or knowledge about how to engage. Most of us live with multiple organizing principles, and situational factors can drive one of them to the fore, suppressing all the others. As we adapt to current expectations, we risk losing a part of ourselves as it atrophies or fails to evolve.

Learning to juggle competing organizing principles may be the fundamental challenge of maturing. I'm more comfortable with some of my own behaviors than others. Not helping those passengers anxious about missing their next flight and focusing on my work instead feels okay to me. On the other hand, I am concerned that my preoccupation with my research distracts me when supervising residents in clinic. When they tell me about sick patients they've just seen, and I'm thinking about my other work or responding to e-mails and phone calls from my research team while they talk—which is sort of like texting while driving—I risk missing important information. Although I remain open to engaging with residents, there is limited opportunity during clinical presentations, as they rattle off lab values and physical exam findings and I nod my head, so my attention can wander. I've found the best way to combat the multitasking is to turn off my cell phone, and to go into the exam room and meet the patient, which pulls me back into the present moment.

Thinking about other work when I should be thinking about patient care may sound quaint compared to all the other things that can distract. Like everyone else, doctors can have affairs; financial problems;

festering resentment toward a colleague, neighbor, or spouse; a sports, gambling, or stock market preoccupation; and the list goes on. But, in truth, it doesn't really matter what's distracting you if it results in a missed diagnosis or erroneous treatment plan.

A line is crossed, however, from competing to conflicting when, as noted earlier, an organizing principle is not only a potential distraction but is irreconcilable with healing. There have been countless news stories of physicians who get rich doing unnecessary procedures, prescribing medications people don't need because drug companies reward them, and billing for services they didn't render, sometimes to the point of criminality. One hospital in Chicago was paying homeless people to come in for cardiac procedures, and then billing Medicare. It may be that the physicians engaged in these activities were never healers to begin with. They were just in it for the money, whatever the consequences. However, I suspect it's not so straightforward in many instances. Surely there are physicians who care about their patients and want the best for them while also wanting to earn more. They may choose lucrative subspecialties, move into positions of leadership, or start new businesses intent on also doing what is best for their patients, but they are drawn into a culture of wealth, based on the neighborhoods they live in and who they mingle with. Conversely, physicians who choose less lucrative specialties may discover that higher earnings are more important to them than they thought, as the work itself doesn't fulfill them as expected, so they see a higher patient volume in a shorter time.

The more organizing principles you have that compete with or conflict with healing, the more likely the healing impulse is to get snuffed out like a candle. Simon is the only person I know for whom healing seems to be the only organizing principle or, at least, the overwhelmingly dominant one. He embodies the ethicist William F. May's description of the fully actualized physician as one who "eats to heal, drives to heal, reads to heal, comforts to heal, rebukes to heal, and rests to heal." Before he had a stroke in his early 80s, he arrived at his office at the military medical school where he worked as a civilian faculty member every weekday morning at about 4:30. His door was always open, signaling to students, faculty, and staff that if they wanted to talk, they could just stop by. Given that it was a military setting, people would drop in early before heading off to their assigned duties. Whatever else he was doing, responding to their concerns always took priority. This mindset was no different in his clinical practice or outside the office in his personal relations. And yet, his phone didn't ring off the hook. One reason, I suspect, is that Simon always gives you his fullest attention, which means he notices even the subtlest inconsistencies and asks about them. The effect is that it compels people to reflect on their own patterns of thinking and behavior, which is challenging. Being a healer 24/7 may sound exhausting, but Simon has always struck me as the calmest, most centered person I've met, probably because he doesn't have a competing organizing principle like making money or achieving stature to distract him.

Becoming a Healer

Since it is not possible to become a healer if you are not engaged with the people you care for, and engaging with boundary clarity is not a skill but a way of being, it can't be learned in the same way you learn a task. In fact, it's the other way around: engaging with boundary clarity is a natural state that you fall into when you are able to free yourself from fear of vulnerability, lack of trust in your own basic goodness, and the tendency to make assumptions about people. What's left is a receptive, open-minded person. In lieu of taking off the shackles, however, physicians who don't engage adopt countless rationalizations for why engaging with patients isn't possible: not enough time during the visit, a lack of incentives, patients are too demanding, charting is too distracting, and so on. If you are going to succumb to those externalities you are, in effect, throwing in the towel on much of your life, given the commitment you have made to your career, the amount of time you'll spend doing it, and the global effect that holding people at a distance has on your life.

If you do not succumb, however, you may have to contend with inner challenges: that you are not sure how to engage with people or what it even means; that engaging seems frightening or inappropriate in the doctor-patient encounter because you are not clear on how to engage without crossing personal boundaries; that you can't stop being a snob or, at least, judgmental; and that you are too preoccupied with other things in your life to connect with most of your patients.

Where to start? The foundation has to be self-trust: the belief in your own basic goodness—that while you may at times be clumsy or distracted and say or do the wrong thing, you don't intentionally harm anyone (except, hypothetically, in self-defense). Define yourself by your own basic goodness, and live by it. If you are basically good, then all else is forgivable. You can acknowledge your faults because they are forgivable. There is profound strength in believing you are basically good, as it gives you the confidence to grow and change rather than just play it safe all the time and keep people at a distance.

What then, is basic goodness? As the term indicates, it's basic: can you honestly say to yourself, reflecting on how you live your life, that you don't knowingly inflict harm? If you learned that something you were doing harms others, would you make an all-out effort to stop? If you saw someone about to be harmed and you could intercede without excessive risk to yourself, would you do so? Think about your intentions, particularly in one-on-one interactions. Good people seek to make the world a better place for others, not as an abstraction, but in individual encounters.

If you have this self-trust, then you can face your shortcomings without feeling like a failure. This enables a process that is essential to personal growth: when you feel uncomfortable about how you may have handled an interaction, rather than suppressing the incident out of a sense of shame, you can look at it objectively, knowing that it is not a referendum on you. You are a fine person, even if you fell short of what the other person needed and you could have offered. That mindset is the only way to take the risk of opening up to engage and then, through experience, to recognize boundaries—yours and your patients'. The alternative is feeling like a failure or denying that you might have erred, which leads not to growth but to stagnation.

Conversely, if you cannot feel confident that you are a "good egg"— for instance, if you are gratified seeing others squirm or would rather make a buck than do what's right for a patient, then you have a problem. It's time to step away from responsibility for vulnerable people and, ideally, find someone you trust with whom you can work through your issues.

If you can trust in your own basic goodness, you will no longer avert your eyes from your patients' struggles out of a sense that you have little personal to offer, rigidly fixating on algorithms and clinical guidelines. You will be able to acknowledge that blindly following these without knowing if they are what your patients really need is not good enough. You will want to ask questions to determine your patients' true needs: What are the implications for them of undergoing a recommended surgery or starting a new medication given what else is going on with them? Are they ready? Is it going to derail their life because of something you don't know about? Do they need a few weeks to think about it?

A second essential component of becoming a healer is self-care. Think of those instructional videos on planes that remind passengers to put on their own oxygen masks first before putting them on their children. It's a useful but oversimplified metaphor, as "physician, first heal thyself" isn't a two-step process. Data on medical student and physician depression and burnout indicate that a large proportion of physicians are not okay—they aren't getting enough oxygen—but they still have to show up for school or work every day. So self-care has to happen concurrently and continuously throughout your training and life. Self-care, of course, has to start with survival, which during medical school means finding a way to pass all the tests required to advance to the next level. Skipping class so that I could study on my own instead of wasting time in lectures I couldn't follow enabled me to survive. It was part of my self-care.

If passing tests is the foundation of survival in the first few years of medical training, organizational skills are the sine qua non of internship and residency. I needed a method for keeping track of everything as patients rolled in and out, labs and test results poured in, consultations had to be set up, and families were waiting to talk with me while, at the same time, my pager kept buzzing as nurses wanted orders, my senior resident had something they needed me to do, and I was about to go on rounds with the attending. After trial and error, I adopted a system learned from one of my chief residents that combined a daily "scut" sheet, a little black notebook organized just so, and rules for how to prioritize ordering consultations, discharging patients ready to go home, and so forth. Once I had the system down pat, I wasn't fazed by even the busiest service. It counted as self-care because now I could cope. If you've figured out how to pass tests and function in a busy clinical setting, you've cleared the equivalent of "basic needs" in Abraham Maslow's hierarchy: you're safe (no one is going to kick you out), and you have enough mastery over your duties to rest and eat.

Another essential element of self-care is friendship. I can think of several people who affirmed me while I was in medical school, each in different ways. One, a classmate who was also struggling, had a wicked sense of humor about our situation. He would do hilarious impressions of some of our teachers and administrators who had immense power over us, unmasking their insincerity. Another friend couldn't have been less like me: he was tall and handsome, excelled academically, and partied a lot. Yet he also seemed to value spending time with me, showing great warmth and opening up in ways that he couldn't with others. Being valued by someone so successful and popular helped me feel less freakish. There was also a graduate student I met in first-year biochemistry who, like me, was a fish out of water. We became good friends who had dinner together quite often. She married a close college friend of mine whom she met through me, and thirty years later we are still in touch. And above all, there was Simon, whom I didn't see often but spoke with at least once a week.

These two core components, trust in our own basic goodness and self-care, including the right sorts of friendships, give us the courage and confidence to change and grow. To become healers we must experience relationships that are engaged and characterized by clarity around personal boundaries. They are a training ground for becoming a healer.

Healers are open to engaging with clarity about boundaries in nearly every encounter, giving people an invaluable resource to turn to when they are in distress. I say "nearly" because if their openness is met with degradation or abuse, they'll retreat. However, they don't lash back, recognizing that the other person's bad behavior is coming from some place they can't fathom and that the only sensible thing to do is to keep them at a distance. But they also don't stop being healers, because engaging respectfully and positively is who they are.

Why Health Care and the World Need Healers More Than Anything

We're living in a world in which influential public figures showcase nastiness and ruthless competitiveness as a badge of merit. Loneliness is rampant. Drug addiction and suicide are major public health problems. People are deeply polarized. Fear and hate are driving mass behavior, exploited by individuals whose organizing principles are seeking power and advancing their careers. Fortunately, there are also a lot of healers out there. Healing as an organizing principle stands out from the others in that it is the foundation of a civilized society. Specifically, those individuals, whatever their profession, who care about and look out for their families, neighbors, and—perhaps most important—strangers, are the most valuable assets a community has. In private spaces, in one-on-one encounters, they help people turn away from the mob and listen to their inner selves. By affirming others as individuals, healers enable those who depend on ideology for identity and feelings of self-worth to open themselves to reasoned discourse, because they trust that they will not be judged for changing their minds.

Medicine is a field where being a healer is a professional necessity, as technical competence combined with no more than an amiable persona is inadequate in many patient care situations. The repercussions of illness extend into nearly all aspects of life: work, sex, caregiving, sleep, emotional well-being, and financial security, to name a few. Facing these challenges alone exacerbates fear and a sense of isolation. If a physician does not engage, they may be present and pleasant, but the patient is still alone. While as a doctor you can't solve all the problems that arise with illness, you can be the one who acknowledges them; who doesn't look away when your patient struggles; who, because you are fully engaged, will ask the questions that need to be asked; and who, because you are clear about boundaries, can keep the interaction on track. And with engagement comes real human attachment. At a personal level, you get to be yourself all day, with the added satisfaction of seeing how that makes you a unique asset to patients you no longer just take care of but care about.

Questions for Reflection and Discussion

1. How important is it to you that people meeting you for the first time in the personal sphere learn that you are a physician or a physician in training? If it is important, why do you think that is?

2. Have you observed or do you know someone whom you would describe as a healer? What are that person's characteristics? For instance, is it a way of relating to people that lifts spirits? Being particularly nonjudgmental and kind? Do you know a physician who has these characteristics?

3. What do you think are your organizing principles? Specifically, what do you find yourself prioritizing in your life, on a day-to-day basis, that others and other activities must yield to? What sorts of things would you feel bad about if you didn't do?

4. How important is it to you that others can turn to you if they are having a hard time and that they feel comfortable doing so? Can you think of people in your life who do confide in you about personal matters? If so, how have you responded? Do you think you were helpful to them? If so, how important was that to you?

5. Have you ever been the direct supervisor of people over whom you have significant authority, whether they are medical students, interns, or individuals outside of the medical field? Did you see your role mainly as telling them what to do or helping them to succeed? Have you encountered situations in which they were struggling or doing poorly? If so, how have you responded?

Introduction

"Idealism." In: English Oxford Dictionaries.com. Retrieved October 9, 2018, from https://en.oxforddictionaries.com/definition/us/idealism.

Kohn LT, Corrigan JM, Donaldson MS, eds. *To Err Is Human: Building a Safer Health System*. Washington, DC: National Academy Press; 2000.

May WF. Code and covenant, or philanthropy and contract? In: Reiser SJ, Dyck AJ, Curran WJ. *Ethics in Medicine: Historical Perspectives and Contemporary Concerns*. Cambridge, MA: MIT Press; 1977:65–76.

Weiner SJ. Contextualizing medical decisions to individualize care: lessons from the qualitative sciences. *J Gen Intern Med* 2004;19:281–285.

Weiner SJ, Schwartz A. Contextual errors in medical decision making: overlooked and understudied. *Acad Med* 2016;91:657–662.

Weiner SJ, Schwartz A. *Listening for What Matters: Avoiding Contextual Errors in Health Care*. Oxford: Oxford University Press; 2016.

Weiner SJ, Schwartz A, Sharma G, et al. Patient-centered decision making and health care outcomes: an observational study. *Ann Intern Med* 2013;158(8): 573–579.

Weiner SJ, Schwartz A, Weaver F, et al. Contextual errors and failures in individualizing patient care: a multicenter study. *Ann Intern Med* 2010; 153(2):69–75.

Chapter 1. Physician or Technician?

Buber M. *I and Thou*. Translated by Ronald Gregor Smith. New York: Scribner; 1958.

Greene A. Why children ask "why." Retrieved July 27, 2019, from https://www.drgreene.com/qa-articles/why-children-ask-why.

Chapter 2. Healing Interactions

Halpern J. *From Detached Concern to Empathy: Humanizing Medical Practice*. New York: Oxford University Press; 2001.

Peabody FW. The care of the patient. *JAMA* 1927;88(12):877–882.

Remen, RN. Interviewed in *The New Medicine*, PBS documentary, March 29, 2006. Directed by Muffie Meyer. Produced by Middlemarch Films and Twin Cities Public Television. Segment on YouTube, https://www.youtube.com /watch?v=AsBxYxvbO-A.

Weiner SJ, Auster S. From empathy to caring: defining the ideal approach to a healing relationship. *Yale J Biol Med* 2007;80:123–130.

Chapter 3. Your Personal Journey

Weiner SJ. Learning medicine with a learning disability: reflections of a survivor. *Acad Med* 2002;77(7):709.

Chapter 4. Overcoming Judgmentalism

Soon CS, Brass M, Heinze H-J, Haynes J-D. Unconscious determinants of free decisions in the human brain. *Nature Neuroscience* 2008;11:543.

Chapter 5. Engaging with Boundary Clarity

Buckwalter JG. The good patient. *N Engl J Med.* 2007 Dec 20;357(25):2534–2535.

"Demeanor." In: Merriam-Webster.com. Retrieved July 26, 2019, from https://www.merriam-webster.com/dictionary/demeanor.

Luoma JB, Martin CE, Pearson JL. Contact with mental health and primary care providers before suicide: a review of the evidence. *Am J Psychiatry* 2002 June;159(6):909–916.

"Persona." In: Merriam-Webster.com. Retrieved July 26, 2019, from https://www.merriam-webster.com/dictionary/persona.

Shem S. *The House of God: A Novel.* New York: R. Marek Publishers; 1978.

Chapter 6. Caring

Association of American Medical Colleges (AAMC). *Learning Objectives for Medical Student Education: Guidelines for Medical Schools.* https://members.aamc.org/eweb/upload/Learning%20Objectives%20for%20Medical%20Student%20Educ%20Report%20I.pdf. Last accessed February 1, 2019.

Berkson G. Social responses to abnormal infant monkeys. *Am J Phys Anthrop* 1974;38:583–586.

"Care." In: English Oxford Dictionaries.com. Retrieved October 4, 2018, from https://en.oxforddictionaries.com/definition/care.

Chapman EN, Kaatz A, Carnes M. Physicians and implicit bias: how doctors may unwittingly perpetuate health care disparities. *J Gen Intern Med* 2013;28:1504–1510.

"Compassion." In: English Oxford Dictionaries.com. Retrieved October 1, 2018, from https://en.oxforddictionaries.com/definition/compassion.

"Compassion." In: Merriam-Webster.com. Retrieved October 1, 2018, from https://www.merriam-webster.com/dictionary/compassion.

Dosa DM. A day in the life of Oscar the cat. *N Engl J Med* 2007;357:328–329.

"Empathy." In: Burchfield RW, ed. *A Supplement to the Oxford English Dictionary.* Vol. 1. London: Oxford University Press; 1972:936.

Glaser BG, Straus AL. *The Discovery of Grounded Theory: Strategies for Qualitative Research.* Chicago: Aldine; 1967.

Hallet JP, Pelle A. *Animal Kitabu.* New York: Random House; 1968.

Halpern J. *From Detached Concern to Empathy: Humanizing Medical Practice.* New York: Oxford University Press; 2001.

Halpern J. What is clinical empathy? *J Gen Intern Med* 2003;18:670–674.

Kelm Z, Womer J, Walter JK, Feudtner C. Interventions to cultivate physician empathy: a systematic review. *BMC Med Educ* 2014;14:219.

Physician burnout: It's not you, it's your medical specialty. Sara Berg for AMA Wire. August 3, 2018. Retrieved October 4, 2018, from https://wire.ama -assn.org/life-career/physician-burnout-it-s-not-you-it-s-your-medical -specialty.

Siebenaler JB, Caldwell DK. Cooperation among adult dolphins. *J Mamm* 1956;37:126–128.

Skosireva A, O'Campo P, Zerger S, Chambers C, Gapka S, Stergiopoulos V. Different faces of discrimination: perceived discrimination among homeless adults with mental illness in healthcare settings. *BMC Health Serv Res* 2014;14:376.

Smedley BD, Stith AY, Nelson AR, eds. *Unequal Treatment: Confronting Racial and Ethnic Disparities in Healthcare.* Washington, DC: National Academy Press; 2003.

"Spiderman" granted French citizenship after rescuing child from Paris balcony. Saskya Vandoome, Samantha Beech and Ben Westcott for CNN. May 28, 2018. Retrieved October 4, 2018 from https://www.cnn.com /2018/05/28/asia/paris-baby-spiderman-rescue-intl/index.html.

Trollope-Kumar K. Do we overdramatize family physician burnout?: NO. *Can Fam Physician* 2012;58:731–733,735–737.

Weiner SJ. Contextualizing medical decisions to individualize care: lessons from the qualitative sciences. *J Gen Intern Med* 2004;19:281–285.

Weiner SJ, Auster S. From empathy to caring: defining the ideal approach to a healing relationship. *Yale J Biol Med* 2007;80:123–130.

Chapter 7. Making Medical Decisions

Binns-Calvey AE, Malhiot A, Kostovich CT, LaVela SL, Stroupe K, Gerber BS, Burkhart L, Weiner SJ, Weaver FM. Validating domains of contextual factors essential to patient-centered care using qualitative methods. *Acad Med* 2017;92(9):1287–1293.

Haynes RB, Devereaux PJ, Guyatt GH. Clinical expertise in the era of evidence-based medicine and patient choice. *ACP J Club* 2002;136:A13.

Weiner SJ. From research evidence to context: the challenge of individualizing care. *ACP J Club* 2004Nov–Dec;141:A11.

Chapter 8. Healers Are Realists

Never doubt that a small group of thoughtful, committed citizens can change the world; indeed, it's the only thing that ever has. In: Quote Investigator. Retrieved July 24, 2019, from https://quoteinvestigator.com/2017/11/12 /change-world.

Chapter 9. Physician or Technician? (Revisited)

Association of American Medical Colleges (AAMC) News. Medical school affordability and student aid. https://news.aamc.org/for-the-media/article /affordability-and-student-aid. October 23, 2018.

Don't Quit Your Day Job (DQYDJ). Individual income percentile calculator: statistics in 2018. https://dqydj.com/income-percentile-calculator. November 20, 2018.

Medscape Physician Compensation Report 2018. https://www.medscape.com /slideshow/2018-compensation-overview-6009667?faf=1. April 11, 2018.

Chapter 10. Healing as an Organizing Principle

Maslow AH. A theory of human motivation. *Psychological Review* 1943;50(4):370–396.

Page numbers in *italics* refer to figures.

catheters, inserting in necks, 56
character traits: of patients, attributing behavior to, 77, 135–36; of physicians, and discontent with job, 163
chasing diagnoses, 129–30
chasing wealth, 150, 177
chelation therapy, 46
children: dealing with abuse of, 78–80; intervening to protect, 79; spanking of, 29–30, 72
chronic conditions, caring for patients with, 28–29
clinical state, in medical decision making, 129, 132, 135
communication with patients: classes teaching, 38–39; about end-of-life care, 106–7; healers as establishing, 169; models of, in medical schools, 32–33. *See also* engagement with others; healing interactions
communities, tackling problems of, 150–52
compartmentalization of life, 54
compassion, definition of, 110
competence and confidence, 168
conflict, interpersonal, dealing with, 64
conformity: drawbacks of, 61; pressure for, 24–25
connection with others. *See* engagement with others
constant comparison, 127
context: in medical decision making, 131–32, 133–37, 138–39; probing for, 136, 137
contextual errors, 10–11, 158–59
contextual factors, 136–37
contextualizing care, 11–12, 37–38, 136–39
contextual red flags, 134–35, 136
Conway, LaMenta, 150–53
coping mechanisms, of medical students, 170
crying, dealing with, 106
cultural competence, 126
culture of medical schools and residency, 54, 57, 67
curiosity: definition of, 69; education and, 62; importance of, 61–65,

69–71; of medical students, 119–20; patient context in medical decision making and, 136; about patients, 9–12, 47–48, 69–70; about world, 22, 23–24

decision making, medical: context and preferences in, 133–39; types of information to consider in, 129–33, *133*
demeanor, 93, 102
depersonalization and burnout, 117–19
detached professionalism: engaged interaction compared to, 84–89, *86, 87*; example of, 40; fear of engagement and, 72; reasons for, 105–6; of technicians, 70–71
diagnoses, chasing, 129–30
"difficult," labeling patients as, 41–47, 89–90
discontent with job: analysis of, 163–64, 165; engagement and, 164; leaving positions and, 166; productivity requirements and, 157–58, 164–65
discrimination in health care, 123–24
disengagement: from others, reasons for, 12–13; from patients, intentional, 90
disrespect, behaving with, 65
distractions, dealing with, 176–77
distrust and suspicion, vibe of, from patients, 97
doctor and patient: bridging divide between, 2, 8–9; negative interactions of, 169–70; stepping outside conventions of encounters between, 68–69. *See also* boundary clarity, interpersonal; engagement with others; patients; physicians
Doctors Without Borders (MSF), work for, 143–46
"drug seeking," labeling patients as, 12, 42, 82, 101
duration of visits: constraints on, 157–60; contextualizing care and, 38; engagement and, 36–37, 85; obtaining psychosocial information and, 48

emergency medical technician, work as, 1–2

emotional issues: of caring for elderly or persons with chronic conditions, 28–29; healing interactions and, 36; in medical school, 26–27; in personal sphere, 95–96; self-awareness of, 102; trauma, repackaging and inflicting on others, 29–33; ways of dealing with, 27–28; of young adulthood, 5. *See also* trust in others

emotional labor, 28

empathy, 110–12, 113–14, 121–22

end-of-life care, talking about, 106–7

engagement with others: advice related to, 6; attachment, fulfillment, and, 29; becoming healer and, 178–82; building rapport compared to, 38–41; caring and, 41–42; contextualizing care and, 11–12, 37–38; curiosity and, 22, 23–24, 47–48; description of, 3, 83–84; detached professionalism compared to, 84–89, 86, 87; discontent with job and, 164; equality and, 31–32; experience of, 173, 175–76; importance of, in medicine, 182–83; link between caring and, 115–21; motivation for, 116; openness to, 31–32, 36, 72, 94, 103–4; patient context in medical decision making and, 135; in personal sphere, 93–97; physicians as impediments to, 36; in professional sphere, 4–5; purpose of, 78; and reasons for disengagement, 12–13; respect for boundaries and, 36–37; self-trust and, 13; setting and context of, 91–92; time constraints and, 158–60; vulnerability of, 39, 88, 106. *See also* boundary clarity, interpersonal

environment, belief in rising above, 77–78

equality of all people, belief in, 65–66

escapist coping mechanisms of medical students, 170

expectations: of medical school, complying with, 56; of parents, 96; of patients, 84; unrealistic, 141–43

external validation, reliance on, 60, 67

failure, being okay with, 57–61, 66–69

false positives, risk of, 130

families: relationships with, 7–8, 45–46, 64, 75–76; working with, 125, 175–76

fear of patients, 41–42

friendship, self-care and, 181

From Detached Concern to Empathy (Halpern), 40, 111, 113

"From Empathy to Caring" (Weiner and Auster), 40–41

fundamental attribution error, 135–36

Gassama, Mamoudou, 112, 121

genetic potential, belief in rising above, 77–78

Greene, Alan, 23

grounded theory, 126–27

growth, as healer, 101–7, 181–82

Halpern, Jodi, 40, 111, 113

harm to patients: from boundary violations, 86–87, 90–91, 91; from productivity requirements, 157, 164

healers: growth as, 101–7, 181–82; identity as, 168, 169; patients as in need of, 169; as realists, 143–53; in society, 182; technicians compared to, 139, 169–70, 173–74

healing, as organizing principle, 169–78

healing interactions: characteristics of, 3–4; engagement with boundary clarity as, 92–93; fulfillment through, 28; judgmentalism as antithetical to, 77; as mutually nourishing, 34–36; relating in the moment and, 48–49. *See also* engagement with others

hidden curriculum of medical schools, 51

homelessness, interactions with persons experiencing, 123–24

hubris and judgmentalism, 80–81

hypothesis testing, 127

I Am Abel Foundation, 151, 152–53

idealism and disillusionment, 141–42, 144, 155

identity as healer, 168, 169–70

ABOUT THE AUTHOR

Saul J. Weiner, MD, is a professor of medicine, pediatrics, and medical education at the University of Illinois at Chicago (UIC) and deputy director of the Veterans Health Administration's Center of Innovation for Complex Chronic Healthcare, a federally funded research center of excellence. He served as senior associate dean for educational affairs at the University of Illinois College of Medicine, where he oversaw medical education. Along with Alan Schwartz, he founded and directs the Institute for Practice and Provider Performance Improvement (I3PI). Dr. Weiner received his MD from Dartmouth Medical School and completed a combined residency in internal medicine and pediatrics at the University of Chicago; he is board-certified in both disciplines. He was a Robert Wood Johnson Generalist Physician Faculty Scholar and a recipient of a clinician teaching award from the medical students' honor society, Alpha Omega Alpha. His book *Listening for What Matters: Avoiding Contextual Errors in Health Care*, coauthored with Alan Schwartz, received the 2017 American Publishers Award for Professional & Scholarly Excellence (PROSE) in the Biological & Life Sciences from the Association of American Publishers (AAP).